Lorraine Candy is a mother of journalist with over a decade parenting in national newspaper the co-host of the chart-topping l *Midlife*, which features the stories of spirited midlife women and tackles parenting adolescents. Formerly the editor-in-chief of *Sunday Times Style*, *ELLE* and *Cosmopolitan*, she is now focusing full-time on writing.

Praise for *'What's Wrong With Me?'*:

'This comforting memoir will help us all feel less alone as we navigate the emotional turmoil of midlife. It's full of advice and stories to support everyone who needs a bit of reassurance, that it really is all going to be OK and the best is yet to come . . . coz it really is'   Davina McCall, author of *Menopausing*

'Read Lorraine's words, take comfort in them and then equip yourself with the advice she has gathered. Use it to navigate your way through your midlife years. The power of sharing our feelings and experiences and supporting one another cannot be underestimated and that's what this book does. There's magic within these pages'   Jo Whiley, *BBC Radio 2*

'At last, a book that we can all relate to in so many different ways! Lorraine uses her vast experience, both personally and professionally, to educate, reassure and guide us to have the most positive and healthy midlife'

Dr Louise Newson, author of *Menopause*

By the same author:

'Mum, What's Wrong With You?':
101 Things Only Mothers of Teenage Girls Know

'What's Wrong With Me?'

From Unravelling to Reinvention
A Midlife Memoir

LORRAINE CANDY

4th ESTATE • London

4th Estate
An imprint of HarperCollins*Publishers*
1 London Bridge Street
London SE1 9GF

www.4thEstate.co.uk

HarperCollins*Publishers*
Macken House
39/40 Mayor Street Upper
Dublin 1
D01 C9W8, Ireland

First published in Great Britain in 2023 by 4th Estate
This 4th Estate paperback edition published in 2024

1

A catalogue record for this book is available from the British Library

ISBN 978-0-00-853013-6

This book has been written by Lorraine Candy based on her own
experiences and knowledge; the advice in it should be used to
complement, and not as a substitute for, professional advice.

Set in Granjon by Palimpsest Book Production Ltd,
Falkirk, Stirlingshire

Printed and bound in the UK using
100% renewable electricity at CPI Group (UK) Ltd

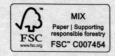

MIX
Paper | Supporting
responsible forestry
FSC™ C007454

This book contains FSC™ certified paper and other controlled sources
to ensure responsible forest management.

For more information visit: www.harpercollins.co.uk/green

For James, Sky, Grace, Henry, Mabel and Pixel

Contents

Preface: How to Use This Book

How did I get here? Did it happen all at once, in a day, over-night? While I was watching *Top of the Pops*? Did it ambush me suddenly from behind? Who is that in the mirror? I'm not familiar with *her*. Was I distracted when I was informed about this – looking at my phone maybe? Why did no one tell me it was coming? Is it a secret? Is it happening to anyone else? None of it makes sense. I must be losing my mind, going mad . . . Who am I? What's wrong with me?

One minute I'm melancholy and meh, the next I am manic and murderous.

I can't remember anything. My mind has gone foggy. Sleep eludes me. My chest is squeezed with panic. I'm fearful of driving and everything makes me cross. Sometimes I hear myself low-level growling with irritation, like Marge Simpson.

That's not normal. I'm a swirly mess of angst and rage, a contrary mix of shame and indignant fury. I'm also very tired. I find my door keys in the fridge, address my mum's birthday card to her dog and leave the house for work with mascara on only one eye.

And why is a cloud of hopelessness floating behind me? Why do I keep doing death maths in the post-office queue? I've never felt like this before; it is confusing, illogical and out of character. And it has caught me completely by surprise.

If any of the above sounds familiar to you, you've picked up the right book. You're not alone. There IS something unexpected in the bagging area. But don't despair, don't worry; you're not trapped in this unusual bewilderment forever. More harmonious, more positive times lie ahead; it's just that you have reached the messy middle bit of life and may need help navigating it – some comforting guidance through these unexpected times before being liberated into a new place. Which is where I come in. You'll be glad to see me. I think I know how you got here, because I know you.

My career has been built on understanding the lives of the women of Generation X. From the newspaper journalism I've focused on to the glossy magazines I've edited (*Cosmopolitan*, *ELLE*, *Sunday Times Style*), my world has been your world.

I was there as you hurtled out of your twenties into the panic years of your thirties. I lived through the '90s party years with you (that was fun); through the ambitious days of shoulder-padded career escapades (very Melanie Griffith in *Working Girl*); through Princess Diana's wedding and her funeral; through your forties, your mothering or not mothering; through all the wolf whistling, mansplaining and manspreading. I have interviewed many of your female heroes and met your role models, sat in the corridors of power with the women fighting for your rights and I have even worked for the woman who invented that goddamn phrase 'having it all'.

So, you see, I am woven into the fabric of your Gen-X life. And here we are now, at a new stage of it, the uncomfortable middle bit. The bit that is not for the faint-hearted, the dangerous age. I co-present a podcast about this: *Postcards from Midlife*. And now I have written a book on it, on us, which I hope is an uplifting guide to navigating midlife using all the wisdom and experiences gathered from the brilliant women I have met: those who have gone before us and those who are going through it with us, as well as all the experts supporting us. I hope this book is a pathfinder for women of our generation: that it is a thoughtful, hopefully humorous glimpse into your possible future. It's not a fierce rallying cry, or a to-do list; it's not about being the best you can be or supercharging your second act with newfound ambitions; it's not about reinvention or feeling younger. It's not about menopause and perimenopause, though we do cover that, obviously (it's unavoidable). There will be no *Cosmo*-style quizzes, commandments or rules. I don't have all the answers, but I am here to give you a gentle nudge towards a less overwhelming place, to motivate you by holding a torchlight on a calmer, more positive mindset. I'll share a few ideas for you to mull over as you embrace the privilege of getting older.

Right now, it most likely feels as if you are on your own, straddling who you were and who you might want to be. The Marigold Hotel is a long way off and you're not falling for anything with 'anti-flush technology' written on the label (that just makes your Gen-X rage worse), but here and now you're in a bit of a wobbly and contrary place. Perhaps you feel self-conscious or self-indulgent for even wondering what's wrong with you, but the good news is that you're not alone. And it does get easier and begin to make sense. You'll find your mojo again! Some work must be done – it may involve a little 'wellness waffle', as I used to call it, and a loose plan must be made, but an army of Gen-X women are alongside you and we are all on this adventure together.

The Unravelling

If the car clipped my left side, perhaps just knocking me over gently (if such a thing were possible), then I figured I would get at least three days away from life in my forties. I obviously didn't want any head injuries or facial scars. Looking in the mirror was already a confusing daily ritual; further damage beyond the ever-deepening frown lines would be unhelpful and upsetting.

All I needed was a small bump, enough to warrant an ambulance, with a siren, followed by a short but revitalising stint in a hospital bed. I was desperate for stillness so that I could figure out what the hell was going on, to make sense of this gradual but disturbing emotional unravelling. This odd sense of losing myself. This weird panic. And I needed a moment alone without being ambushed by memories of days gone by. It was all so strange. I had lost the ability to remember the password to my computer, yet the day we first took our toddler to the London Aquarium or the moment my dad gave me away at my wedding more than two decades ago would suddenly pop into my head. Crystal-clear memories, right down to the smells, sounds and even temperatures. This technicolour footage would stop me in my tracks and take my breath away; this 'previous life' kept flooding into my current life, unexpectedly splattering me with melancholy mayhem. It was bewildering. It was as if I was being stalked by the woman I used to be at the stage of life where I had begun to look for signs of who I was now, because I didn't really know. I was baffled and discombobulated by it all at the age of 47.

I'd get to the end of the day and wonder where I had put 'it', not knowing what 'it' was. I had that feeling of continually rooting around in my handbag looking for my keys, fury mounting, but there was never a sense of relief because I never found my keys and each day the search began again. I was sleeping less and catastrophising more.

I kept muttering, 'What's wrong with me?' under my breath. It's a phrase my increasingly independent teenage daughters said to me every time I appeared anyway, in that way teenage girls have of brutally dismissing their mums.

But what *was* wrong with me? Almost everything, it felt like. As well as the surprise of being constantly ambushed by my 'previous life', I had also developed a low level of panic and anxiety. I was either sorrowful all the time or worried all the time or furious all the time, which was not like me. I'm generally quite a perky person. I was also intermittently overwhelmed and exhausted. And I had started to do the death maths – calculating how long I had left in days. I expected to turn round and see the Grim Reaper standing in our kitchen, petulantly tapping his watch like one of my teens waiting for me to give them a lift.

I was in the autumn of my life and, illogically, this was a terrifying realisation.

Running out of time made me suddenly feel trapped by the

small regularity of things. The biscuit tin being put in the same place every day inexplicably tipped me over the edge with indignant rage. 'Why can't it go here?' I would demand, moving it dramatically to some impractical shelf as my perplexed family looked on. 'Or here?' putting it in the dog-food cupboard under the sink and slamming the door. 'Why does it have to belong somewhere, to be in the same place all the time?' I yelled. Maybe I wasn't talking about the tin, maybe I didn't think I belonged here right now? I didn't know where I belonged anymore. Before something went wrong with me, I didn't feel this unpredictable fury. I didn't care where the biscuit tin belonged. I didn't have time to be specific about biscuits. I just ate them.

I had turned into melancholy Ria from TV sitcom *Butterflies*. But how could I be that old? All. Of. A. Sudden.

And out of the blue there were some mornings where I couldn't summon the energy to care about anything. I just wanted to 'drip' around the house all day, as my daughters would say, like a sad midlife goth. Taking clean laundry slowly up and down the stairs. Answering emails with one word.

My WhatsApp chats were now filled with vignettes of other women my age encountering similar confusion, brain fog and unpredictability, all of them asking, 'Is this normal? Am I normal?' or 'Who am I now?'

Women I knew had taken to inexplicably crying in cars after dropping their kids off at various activities. Some were sitting in supermarket car parks for hours 'thinking' rather than going home. None of us knew who we were any more.

Every time I looked in the mirror it took me by surprise. I would suppress a sigh or a 'Good God, what is this now?' shriek. I didn't want to look younger. I wasn't cross about getting physically older; I just didn't know what personality would match my changing face. Maybe I should try a middle parting instead of the lifelong side one (that's how mad I had gone). Perhaps that was who I was now? A woman with a modern middle parting. My teenage daughters said they would rather never go out than go out with a side parting. Would this make me feel more relevant, less invisible? I would have to find some eyebrows, though, to replace these '90s disasters that I'd noted even Kate Moss couldn't pull off these days.

I had started to wander into rooms wondering why I was there. I would spend hours looking for stuff – phones, hair-bands, keys – and raging relentlessly at the behavioural issues of white goods, especially the printer, which our small dog had taken to guarding (there was a Starburst sweet stuck in it that she wanted). Most sentences began with me saying, 'I'm sorry, what was the question?' over and over again, like some absent-minded, daydreaming professor of uselessness.

'You are like a mug without a handle,' a friend told me when I asked her what was wrong with me. What is a mug without a handle for? I wondered. It was dangerously hot, that's for sure. And when I say hot, I mean angry.

So yes, what I desperately needed was a run-of-the-mill 'accident', on the way to Tesco. But I had to be careful to keep my right side – the dishwasher-unloading, packed-lunch-making, lid-putting-back-on, Christmas-card-writing, sock-pairing, WhatsApp-messaging, doing-my-actual-job side – in reasonable working order or it would become even trickier to push on through what I knew instinctively would take some time to fix.

After my fantasy incident, accident, whatever you want to call it, paramedics would take my phone away (hurrah!) and that morning, before stepping off the pavement at exactly the right moment, I would have made sure my underwear was unremarkable. During a recent MRI of my ovaries (these go wrong when they stop working, like ancient attention-seeking

tumble-driers), the female technician had declared my black
M&S knickers 'a bit fancy for day to day'. I apologised to her.
It wouldn't happen again, I promised. What was I thinking?
What was wrong with me?

In less fancy pants, I could lie in my hospital bed and work
out what the hell was going on, repair the glitch in the matrix.
I just needed a small amount of time – and something funny
had happened to time . . . I didn't understand it anymore. The
bit behind me felt endless – so much had happened: childhood,
leaving home at 16, a career, marriage, motherhood, friendships,
pets living and dying, holidays, parties, love affairs, people living
and dying. But the bit in front of me was hurtling towards me
at a terrifying speed. Tomorrow would be gone in a minute,
surely? I felt as if I was about to gingerly open the gate to
sniper alley, the last part of the journey where anything could
happen, some of it possibly fatal because the end was literally
in sight. This was like living through a darker-than-usual
episode of *Tales of the Unexpected*. My daily soundtrack seemed
to be the lyrics of that '80s tune 'Live It Up': 'Hey, yeah you,
with the sad face' (by a band called, ironically, Mental As
Anything).

Yet nothing extraordinary had happened in my daily life,
nothing dramatic or tragic, to cause this out-of-character,
creeping sadness, this unusual and unexpected sensation of
being lost, of loss, of being alone in a void between yesterday
and tomorrow. It was an unnerving and lonely place to be. And
I seemed to be mourning the end of something I didn't know
had finished, or that had finished suddenly without my permission. This feeling had slipped into my life without me noticing
and now I'd lost my mojo. I couldn't feel hopeful or optimistic,
which was unlike me.

How did I get here? I frequently wondered. Where did I
fit in now? I wanted to be back in the then and not in this

now, to pinch my nose like Mr Claypole in *Rentaghost* and reappear walking up the street outside our house pushing the buggy with one of my little girls in it and holding the warm hand of my son on the way back from school or sitting on the tube to work, clutching my first coffee of the day, enjoying that Monday-morning feeling of being competent, busy, relevant and needed. Of belonging. I didn't want to be over halfway through; it felt so unfair.

Which is why I had started to fantasise about a minor accident so that I could go to hospital for some uninterrupted stoppage, where I would patiently and logically think about all this malarkey. I would rediscover my positivity. I would rest, find my ability to sleep again and I would follow the advice they give you when you are drowning in the sea: stop thrashing about and turn to lie on your back. I needed to lie on my back, and then I wouldn't get dragged under (I feared being dragged under the most). Lying on my back, floating through all these feelings, surely I would be able to work out exactly what was wrong with me? Then I could set about finding what I had lost. Probably the most important thing I owned: my identity.

2

The Creeping Sadness

It all started with the creeping sadness. I was around 47. I announced it in a piece I wrote for *ELLE* when I was 10 years into my editorship of the magazine. For the first time in my life I was physically anxious, and out of the blue I began to have panic attacks. The ground would feel like it was moving beneath me, and I couldn't breathe as a sense of impending doom engulfed me. Something was pressing down on my chest and I would begin to sweat.

This article was intended to be a piece about taking up boxing. Exercise was saving me, I wrote, from being woken up almost every night at 2 a.m. covered in sweat, my head filled with a dark, unknown fear. Exercise, I argued, was helping me grapple with this new demon that seemed to be stopping me from breathing easily; it was holding me together as I felt like I was unravelling. It was perplexing and I viewed all these new thoughts and emotions as a problem to solve.

I told my friend Caroline on WhatsApp that I thought I was going mad. I recalled my mum telling me about a great-aunt who had schizophrenia and I assumed there was a genetic possibility of instability, or even insanity. I was spending an increasing amount of time trying and failing to calm down.

In the chat about my impending lunacy, Caroline told me it was probably something to do with doing too much too fast for such a long period of time.

After all, I had worked full-time at a manic pace for three decades, and I had had four children in 10 years, the last at 43. Obviously I was fully aware that I wasn't working on the frontline of a war zone or saving lives in A&E, so my stress should have been manageable, I reasoned. I was just a failure at managing it.

Maybe you've just broken your brain with all that effort, Caroline suggested. Maybe I have early-onset dementia, I wondered. I had, after all, got into the car at one point and forgotten which side of the road I was supposed to be driving on; terrified, I had to go back indoors to ask my husband, and the teens looked at me as if all their notions had been confirmed. 'What is wrong with you?' one of them asked, mildly disgusted by her mum's consistent failure to be a normal person and furious about someone else having an issue that may require attention.

Sometimes over the next couple of years I would occasionally wake up screaming or gasping in the middle of the night. 'Not to be dramatic', as my adolescents would say, but I found this a little frightening. These night terrors would grip me like a torturer. This wasn't normal. Lights out, for me, had always been like a general anaesthetic; sleeping was one of my superpowers. I handled stress well. I was healthy. I was, like most women of my generation, 'a coper'. Slightly melodramatic, maybe, but generally a 'push-on-through' sort. Besides, life was good and I was grateful for that, so why was I not coping?

11

I just carried on as normal at work, fuelled by a bit of extra coffee and powered by a lack of patience with everybody and everything that had reached record levels. Though I did begin to remember the days when my own mum had seemed very out of sorts when I was a teenager, which would have made her about the same age as I was now. I came home from my summer internship at the *Cornish Times* paper one day, aged 16, and she had painted the garden fence black around our bungalow, which was all a bit *League of Gentlemen*. She once threw our tea at the patio windows and occasionally met me after work to tell me she really couldn't see the point of any of it – life, anything.

One morning on the way to my office I stepped out of my front door and froze on the spot. I couldn't catch my breath, a thin layer of sweat sat on my skin and I felt as if the world was coming towards me at 100 miles an hour. The ground was moving like water, and I was extremely nauseous. Perhaps I was having my first ever grown-up asthma attack, I thought as I struggled to breathe.

Another day I got to work and walked straight past the door to the glossy magazines lobby. I suddenly felt over-whelmed and knew I was too out of sorts to go in, too bonkers to face my team. So I walked around the block several times, up and down Carnaby Street, until I was calm enough to enter a building I had happily worked in for years. This happened a few times. Perhaps I had a brain tumour, I thought, and this was affecting me in odd ways. Pressing down on my 'normality' and switching me into this new, unbalanced individual, one I kept secret from colleagues because I had so much to do; a whole career as an organised and successful individual seemed to be at stake. I tried hard to work around my little problem, writing everything down so I wouldn't forget things, going through lists again and again, double checking everything, relying heavily on my brilliant millennial assistants. A swan on the water, with my legs furiously kicking underneath.

I 'revealed' the creeping sadness by writing about it, which meant I could cloak it in a cape of humour and it became a sort of light-hearted joke. I was foraging for a solution by dreaming up features on it for the magazine I was editing. And besides, self-care and looking after your mental health were becoming buzzwords at this point in journalistic history, so it was OK, I wasn't an anomaly in tending to this situation. I wasn't being self-indulgent in trying to sort it out.

'How's the creeping sadness today?' my colleagues and friends would ask with care. 'Fine,' I would reply, 'no death maths this morning on the road towards turning 50.' Every now and again my empathetic deputy, Lotte, would suggest I walk round the block for some fresh air. I was also running alongside the boxing.

All the while I just kept looking for reasons for how I was feeling that made sense to me. Maybe the insomnia was causing all this panic and fear, I concluded; the night sweats, the dizziness and the rushing sounds in my ears. It was a cycle, a chain to be broken. I had an even better theory: perhaps years of cumulative cortisol (the stress hormone) had built up in my small body (I am only five foot two) and now it was at a level so toxic that it was affecting my brain function. A spot of googling disproved this theory and I trudged on like a nuclear power plant about to blow, cracks all over the concrete. It was humiliating, though, to think that perhaps my choice to have a career and four kids was more stress than I could deal with. What a failure, I thought in the darker moments between the sunnier days. My generally OK level of confidence began to dip. My annoyingly excessive amount of energy dissipated. My overwhelming emotion was confusion, followed closely by rage and forgetfulness. I wasn't in a dark place all the time, more a perplexed one. I had been derailed. My late forties were like constantly living in an escape room looking for clues to the exit.

This frustrating feeling was quite a conundrum; it was beating like a drum in the back of my mind, as if the pounding, doom-laden *Jumanji* theme tune were stalking me. Other women sympathised when I mentioned it; some said they felt it too occasionally. None of us could explain it, though.

My life was good otherwise. I was happy with my husband; we had a lovely part-time nanny helping with childcare as we both worked outside the home. I could cope, I was organised and I had the physical energy to deal with any family setbacks. We had enough money. My elderly dad was in and out of hospital 200 miles away in Cornwall, but none of it seemed life-threatening.

The magazine was doing well, even though the days of print were clearly numbered. I had won awards. A book deal was in the offing. I had a column in a national newspaper. Our school holidays on the beach in my home county of Cornwall soothed my soul. I was grateful every day, especially that my children seemed happy and were healthy. I felt so lucky to be where I was, coming from where I came from, my ordinary background. I wasn't dissatisfied and I didn't look around me wanting what others had. What I had was enough, and that is a powerful thing to be able to say. And yet something was 'off'.

One late-summer afternoon I was walking home from the tube after work in a complete fog. I felt as if someone was kneeling on my chest and I really couldn't see the point of anything I was doing; it was the oddest, deadest feeling. In my head there just seemed no reason for me to be here. This dark feeling of imminent danger was illogical but seemed perfectly sensible inside my head. I was too messy for the normal life around me, I thought. I was jangly; the creeping sadness had turned into an overwhelming sense of something really bad about to happen and I had no control over it. I got to the corner of our road and realised I was in tears – they were just pouring down my face. If I was going to feel like this forever, it was hardly worth it. It was such a strange emotion; a new emotion for me. What the hell was going on?

Still, I didn't join the dots. I just ignored the expanding tendrils of anxiety. 'Get a grip' was my daily motto. I often said it out loud and told my young team if I were to write a self-help book it would be called that. But I was clinging to a ledge, and the sky was closing in on me. I was getting up earlier and earlier to do the things on my list that I knew I had to get out of the way before the day started, because stuff was taking me so much longer to accomplish.

Not going mad

In the end, enough was enough: I went to the GP. 'Go before the wheels come off,' an older friend advised me. I had to sort out this brain tumour/dementia/depression. The first GP I saw, a friendly middle-aged man, asked what I wanted. 'To feel better,' I said, after we'd established there was nothing physically wrong with me bar a low iron count (which explained why my hair was getting thinner) and a sudden severe shellfish allergy (which no one could explain). 'Would antidepressants help?' he replied. He wasn't unsympathetic, but he couldn't explain why I had forgotten which side of the road to drive on or why, when I sat down on the sofa to rest for a few minutes in the afternoon, inexplicably exhausted, I would wake up four hours later.

No, I said; antidepressants may work for some people, but I didn't think they were the answer here. Medication felt like a sticking plaster. I asked if it was something to do with the menopause, because the other gruesome thing I was enduring was horrifically heavy periods. I was using tampons big enough for an elephant and wearing giant nappy-style sanitary pads, all of which had to be changed hourly. This was humiliating and debilitating at the same time. But the GP said I was too young at 47. He made an appointment for me with the practice's young female doctor. 'She'll know more,' he added. Why? I wanted to ask. Just because she has ovaries? Surely you are all trained the same? Women are 51 per cent of the UK population – should a male GP not know about this kind of thing?

When I saw the female doctor she said we could try hormone replacement therapy (HRT) if I felt that strongly about not taking antidepressants. Which I did; I'd done some research on this and felt my symptoms were not related to depression, and several women I knew had been prescribed antidepressants – for some they were a godsend, but for others they changed the quality of their lives for the worse.

But the HRT prescription I asked my GP for made no difference. (When I finally got the right prescription privately later on from the country's leading menopause expert she was perplexed by the initial dose I had been given by the NHS. It was such a small dose it wouldn't have helped a perimenopausal field mouse.)

I began to talk about what was going on with older friends: some implored me to take the happy pills, but a couple told me – well, whispered to me – about the menopause, handing me books and sending me to websites.

I'd interviewed Davina McCall for *Style* magazine, which I moved to after editing *ELLE*, and we'd become friends. She implored me to go to the GP again and demand an effective HRT prescription, explaining that it was also a medicine that prevented heart disease and osteoporosis. I kept resisting, illogically fearful that I was going down the 'unnatural route', and, as it turns out, I was trusting an NHS system that at that time, in 2017, really knew little about what I, and millions of other women, were experiencing. The system was so uninformed about the health of older women that it was mistakenly prescribing antidepressants, keeping many in a zombie land of feeling nothing. I now know, as a journalist expertly informed on the menopause and perimenopause, that a third of women are mistakenly offered antidepressants by their GP, according to a survey by Dr Louise Newson in 2019,[1] mostly because GPs are not thoroughly trained in dealing with women presenting with symptoms – and also, dare I say it, because of the patriarchal attitude to women's pain. A lot of research has been done on the entrenched gender bias of the medical community. A survey as recent as June 2022 showed medics routinely dismissing debilitating women's health problems like endometriosis and heavy bleeding as 'benign',[2] a term widely used by gynaecologists. I've also heard about this attitude anecdotally from almost all the health experts I have interviewed.

Women really are supposed to endure their pain as they age, rather than seek treatment or be offered relief. A friend told me her GP had said she should not 'make a song and dance' of her dire perimenopause symptoms because it was Mother Nature's way. Another had been advised by her older male GP to take up something calming like needlepoint when she went to see him about her extreme memory loss and insomnia.

The writer Kathy Lette is one of my friends (you meet many writers when you edit glossy magazines); she would often take me and her smart gaggle of girlfriends out. I'd sip my drink alongside impressive women like the magnificent Sarah Brown, Pamela Stephenson and Penny Smith and talk out loud about slowly losing my grip.

'Get the hormones,' Kathy said one night when I had drunk far less than everyone else. By this point I had also developed a weird reaction to alcohol; my body couldn't metabolise it anymore so I could no longer tolerate it, and as anyone who knew me before 2017 will attest, I do like a drink, I do, I do, I do. I'd been to the British Fashion Awards earlier that month, where I'd had a glass of wine, which had made me feel so peculiar I had to go outside, the instant dizziness propelling me like a spinning top down the empty red carpet until I had to rest against a wall. First sleep had gone and now booze – both of my superpowers whipped away! I'd have to hand in my cape if this went on.

Even so, I was ignoring the signs that something was wrong; I was just getting on with it. While some of the women around me, my peers, urged another trip to the GP and costly visits to private hormone clinics, some remained tight-lipped about their experience. One told me to keep quiet 'in case they shift you out at work for someone younger'.

'It's unhelpful to talk about menopause out loud,' she said, and implied what I was going through was very rare. 'You don't get hot flushes anyway,' she said dismissively, and so I silently diagnosed terminal cancer instead.

At this point I began to think the murderous rage I felt 90 per cent of the time could come in useful. After all, this wasn't someone's-left-the-lid-off-the-milk-again rage; this was stab-my-husband-to-death-for-leaving-the-lid-off-the-milk rage. It felt as if the rabbit working the controls in my head had suddenly slumped forward and accidentally leaned on the anger button, pushing the dial up to the max.

My husband was terrified of this new Hulk-style wife. The car took quite a battering (two new tailgates), and I know he contemplated hiding the bread knife. 'Why don't you go for a swim?' he'd say, spotting the early signs of the fury as they built up. The inexplicable rage took me by surprise, but it was the thing every woman my age talked about – it was the universal female experience of midlife, and I felt it was time to harness it.

We're all in this together

Around this time, I was still travelling to the bi-annual catwalk fashion shows for work. They sound so glamorous, don't they? And they really are – so many amazing things to see besides the clothes – but they are also the money roadshow. It was non-stop work on the trail of the advertisers' buck.

At the end of Paris Fashion Week in spring – after four weeks away, on and off, when we usually had flu and a permanent headache, and our partners at home were barely on speaking terms with us, having endured sole childcare and 10 bouts of chickenpox – I and the editor-in-chief of *Marie Claire*, Trish Halpin, would often go out for dinner. Neither of us took the fashion element of our job too seriously. Journalism was our real drive on magazines. And this bonded us.

After one set of particularly gruelling catwalk shows dominated by industry bigwigs explaining the internet to us patronisingly while throwing money at the new breed of fashion journalists called 'influencers', Trish and I had one of our end-of-term dinners. My oestrogen levels must have been OK that night because I managed wine as we offloaded all the horrors our minds and bodies were going through, alongside our work problems.

'Don't laugh, Trish,' I said, 'but I think I've got a brain tumour.'

'Me too,' she replied.

Trish told tales of hurling a Hoover down a hallway in a hotel in a rage, of wondering if motherhood had been worth it. We shared the dark secrets of terrible things we'd done around our children. We put our shame on the table and inspected it. Then we put the bill on expenses; our male bosses could pay for this.

Trish, whom I've known for over 20 years, explained she'd been in therapy for two years because of this lonely sense of being overwhelmed and out of control. He mum had died of cancer just before the birth of Trish's twins and she felt her grief was sometimes contributing to her state of mind. She didn't think there could also be a physical reason behind this change of personality. Neither of us had shared with our friends what was going on so this was the first time we'd talked about it out loud.

We weren't moaning, though; we were contemplating the future based on life taking a surprising turn. We were looking for the upside. A positive solution.

We laughed until we cried about the rage. 'It's like being a new superhero, isn't it?' we agreed: Anger Woman, Rage Girl – she would definitely have fire coming out of her cape and ears. 'I wonder how many other women feel like this?' we asked. It felt so good to share our 'symptoms'. I felt unburdened, as if I wasn't the only busy, curious Gen-X woman trying to untangle this unexpected, knotted knitting bag in my head. We instinctively knew, though, that we weren't alone. Later we discovered that almost every woman over 40 felt elements of this and that every woman under 40 was witnessing it. These symptoms were hardly invisible and definitely not silent. We found out that this was the perimenopause: the evil little sister of the menopause.

For a millisecond we did wonder if it was wise to talk about it in public. After all, the moment a woman talks about her age there's a risk she'll be tossed aside like an iffy-smelling, overripe melon. But then we decided, given that between us we'd edited every magazine on the newsstand bar *Vogue*, we owed it to our Gen-X readers to talk about it out loud. It was unkind not to offer the warmth of the message 'you are not alone' to other women, our readers. We were going to find out what was happening on their behalf. We were both trained journalists – this was our job.

But how could we do it? We knew neither of the publications we worked on at that time (*Marie Claire* and *Sunday Times Style*) would want this kind of story in print. Our mag bosses would tell us advertisers would not want to see stories about 'older' women on the pages of the glossies. We knew we'd be viewed suspiciously for writing about women ageing unless: a) it somehow benefited the beauty/fashion industry by whipping up a fear from which companies could profit (this has been happening to women for years and we know we played into this, for which we apologise); b) the women were J.Lo looking sexy or Madonna being labelled 'desperate' for looking sexy. But if we couldn't write it, we could at least talk about it. So we decided to start a podcast. Everyone had one these days; they were the new black. And if anyone knew what was fashionable, on trend, of-the-moment then it was two women who'd sat through 'the fashions', as we called them, for more than two decades, being paid to predict what was coming next. That was us.

And so *Postcards from Midlife* was born. We kept menopause out of the title because there was so much more to discuss with women at this stage of life. And we also kept that word out of the title because, in all honesty, we wanted to be able to start conversations, not have them shut down immediately by a world that was at that time terrified of the 'M' word.

Over the course of the next three years (as I write) we interviewed every well-known midlife celebrity and every expert on the menopause, perimenopause, HRT and breast cancer in the UK. Download numbers are in the millions and our community is enthusiastically engaged and actively spreading information to other women who need it.

As a result of our growing expertise on midlife women and the wonderful community that has sprung up around our podcast, Trish and I have advised many companies on how to help women in the workplace with symptoms and support. We've also advised beauty brands on how to talk to Gen-X women, reminding them that we didn't all want to look younger. We weren't anti-ageing; we just wanted to look and feel better.

We've advised big corporations on policies to make changes that go beyond turning up the air conditioning in a few rooms (God knows how many times we've told people that hot flushes are often the least of our worries and that not every perimenopausal woman has them).

But most importantly, on the podcast we've heard the stories of women our age who have all, without exception, famous or otherwise, been hit over the head by this surprise feeling of loss – of losing themselves. Physical symptoms aside, they ALL (and I mean ALL) had a vulnerable midlife story to tell. A loss of confidence. A confusion about what was going on. How could a whole generation of women know so little about what was happening to their minds and bodies? Why had the generation before us not told us about this secret life they were leading?

It was an inexplicable lack of knowledge, no doubt partly due to our Western culture's ageist attitude towards females. But by sharing women's 'journeys', as we came to refer to it (because we couldn't find a less millennial word), we were helping those who had become stuck in this sometimes dark and surprisingly rickety place. And best of all, when we talked to guests who were further down the road we discovered that what was over the horizon looked good. The story wasn't a negative one; it reinforced our belief that we weren't moaning or complaining, that older women weren't weaker but simply figuring out what we needed to know to get to the 'new you' bit of us that the science and the anecdotal evidence assured us was possible. 'All good things,' as Olaf the snowman would say in *Frozen*.

What do you need to know?

We've learned so much along the way – much of it, it must be said, an awful indictment of the medical profession's treatment of women as they age. I certainly didn't get the right medical support until I decided to see an expert – Dr Louise Newson – who now runs the world's leading menopause clinic.

I first met her before she had written her two bestselling books, launched an award-winning podcast and set up The Menopause Charity. My quest the day I arrived by train at her Stratford upon Avon clinic was personal and professional, and I was lucky to get an appointment; she now has a huge waiting list and is routinely referred to in the press as the menopause specialist to the stars!

I was 49 by this point and deep into my perimenopause: the 10 or so years before the actual menopause, which on average occurs around age 51 in the UK; it is dated from a year after the last day of your last period.

During perimenopause two of your hormones (oestrogen and progesterone) may fluctuate wildly, and because oestrogen is like petrol for the brain and body, when it disappears the physical and mental ripple effects can be hugely debilitating. There are at least 40 symptoms of perimenopause, and they range from tinnitus and joint aches to extreme anxiety, depression and even psychosis. It is different for everyone, and your hormone levels vary daily, which is why there is no one test to find out if you are perimenopausal (don't ever be persuaded to pay for one). Diagnosis is given by joining up the dots of your symptoms and testing for any underlying conditions that may be affecting your health.

I went to see Louise at her wellbeing clinic, a forthright and passionate campaigner for educating GPs and other healthcare professionals better on women's health, as part of a piece I was writing for *Style*'s Spa Special – our annual magazine review of new spas across the globe. It was the only way I could get a piece on the perimenopause (a phrase few journalists had heard of at the time) into the magazine. The Spa Special was the Trojan horse for what I saw as one of the most important features of my career.

Louise and I are now good friends and I'm very familiar with her work, but at that first meeting I kept asking her to clarify facts because I couldn't quite believe what I was hearing. I thought perhaps the insidious grind of the past couple of years of no sleep was affecting my ability to process what seemed like quite an unbelievable back story. She was telling me the story of decades of gaslighting of women by the medical profession.

More than 20 years ago a study called the American Women's Health Initiative had been carried out on women over 63 using a form of hormone replacement therapy no longer prescribed, which linked the treatment with breast cancer.[3] This flawed study, which journalist Kate Muir expertly details in her book *Everything You Need to Know About the Menopause (But Were Too Afraid to Ask)*, set off a chain of events that led to much of the medical profession misinterpreting the results and wrongly believing that HRT should not be given to perimenopausal and menopausal women, because the risk of breast cancer was believed to be too high. After the survey 1 million women in the UK stopped taking HRT.

But for many women replacing the hormones they have lost (oestrogen, progesterone, testosterone) is the only way to ease the symptoms of perimenopause and menopause. Lifestyle changes, like a healthier diet, increased movement and better sleep, can alleviate some symptoms, but the National Institute for Health and Care Excellence (NICE) guidelines now recommend HRT. And the unprecedented over-prescription of antidepressants instead is alarming some doctors in the US, where in 2022 it was found that one in five women between 40 and 59 is now taking them.[4] Senior medics have put this down to other doctors ignoring menopausal symptoms, according to the *Wall Street Journal*.[5]

When you know that the highest rates of suicide for women are among the 45–49-year age group this outdated medical attitude feels even more unforgivable.[6] I have certainly spoken to women who were ready to take their own lives before receiving HRT to help them with their symptoms.

Now, some women may not be able to take HRT. You would need to talk to your specialist about any decision, of course, especially if you have had oestrogen-positive cancers, although some women who have had breast cancer in the past do choose to take it for the health benefits and to improve their quality of life. Also, it can take some time to get the dose right, but for many women body identical HRT is a life saver, a game-changing medicine that boosts their mental and physical health and returns them to their normal selves. Today's body identical natural HRT, and the no-risk vaginal oestrogen pessaries that are usually given to women with vaginal atrophy,[7] have revolutionised the quality of life for many midlifers. It is a scandal that women have been denied hormones on prescription for so long due to a mistake in a medical survey.

Even female GPs are leaving their jobs due to medical sexism around their menopause symptoms – that's how little the profession seems to care about women. A 2020 British Medical Association survey said two out of five women GPs were unable to make changes at work to cope with their symptoms, and a significant number said they would be 'laughed at or ridiculed' by their peers if they spoke about the menopause.[8] So how on earth can we be taken seriously as patients if even female GPs aren't taken seriously?

Perimenopausal women leave jobs, walk away from marriages, abandon families and kill themselves due to these symptoms. I can think of no earthly reason why it is not a better understood chapter in women's health. And, of course, I am viewing this through the lens of my white, heterosexual, privileged life. Black and brown women receive even less support when it comes to their health, and research shows they reach menopause at 49 on average, two years earlier than white women. The LGBTQIA+ community is rarely asked about their needs in this debate either.

It should be noted, too, that the high price of regular three-monthly HRT prescriptions prevents many women from taking it simply because they cannot afford it (though MP Carolyn Harris is campaigning for a one-off yearly prescription payment, rather than expensive monthly repeat prescriptions, given that many women are on HRT for life). And currently only two of our fluctuating or declining hormones are replaced by the NHS in the UK – oestrogen and progesterone – due to the outdated medical complexities of prescribing testosterone (a hormone that helps with debilitating brain fog and concentration). If you want to know more about this, do turn to Kate Muir's book on menopause as it tackles the issues in depth from a medical point of view.

When we interviewed breast-cancer pioneer Professor Michael Baum on the podcast he told us in no uncertain terms that women had been denied HRT as part of the medical profession's ongoing misogyny and the belief that we can simply endure more pain and discomfort than men. He said that on men's cancer wards the prescriptions for pain relief were often much higher than on women's wards. 'I used to go around turning up morphine drips on wards full of women,' he told us.

Attitudes *are* changing, though, as the voices of midlife women are now increasingly being heard. Dr Newson herself has provided free training for more than 30,000 GPs in the UK on the menopause and perimenopause.

As we sat and discussed all this, Dr Newson prescribed me four pumps of oestrogen and one pea-sized amount of testosterone daily. Within a week I felt better. A *week*. The night sweats stopped immediately, the anxiety dissipated and my energy returned. I have not had a panic attack since. I was one of those women for whom menopausal hormone therapy worked instantly. I knew it was a possibility, because so many midlife women who were further down this road had told me it would.

I was physically restored and back in focus instead of blurry round the edges.

I was still lost and confused about my changing identity, but I was grateful that I was privileged enough to have been able to afford this (I paid for a private consultation). I then talked

27

to my NHS GP about prescribing HRT in the correct doses for me based on Dr Newson's prescription and tests.

Back in the room

HRT gradually gave me my sleep back, and that was the root of almost all the other positive changes in my health.

Lack of sleep is a particularly cruel part of the perimenopause story. Night sweats, hot flushes and extreme anxiety can provoke long-term insomnia in women, and often this comes just after you've recovered from the sleepless nights of the childbearing years, which feels like a particularly sick joke.

Kathryn Pinkham, who runs London's Insomnia Clinic, specialises in helping midlife women. On the podcast she told us that once the physical symptoms associated with fluctuating and declining hormones wake you up, it can interrupt your 'sleep drive' to such an extent that the sleeplessness snowballs, and it may take many months to resolve.

Before taking HRT I'd been trapped in a stressful panic around sleep; the night sweats were horrendous, but the anxiety that my mind served up even when there were no sweats was just as difficult to deal with.

Kathryn's advice for all of us going through this is to reduce our fear and stress around not getting enough sleep. Her tips are rooted in cognitive behavioural therapy, which, she says, is the best method for improving sleep patterns (alongside HRT).

When we panic about sleep we usually try to go to bed earlier and get up later, which is a mistake, according to Kathryn. We may also start to associate our beds with troubled nights, meaning that just going into the bedroom can become a cue for poor sleep. She advises that if we wake in the night, we should get up and do something we enjoy, then during the day we should write down exactly what we think will happen if we continue to miss out on sleep so that we're tackling our fears logically in the light of day and getting them out of our heads.

She also told us that quality, not quantity, is important when it comes to sleep and that as we age we get less of the deep sleep that does the most good. So it isn't about staying in bed longer, but more about making the most of the hours we are there and not fretting if we miss a night. It's basically retraining the brain as you go through this stage of life. Antidepressants may help with the panic around insomnia, she says, but they won't cure it. It's about managing the worry about not sleeping during the day.

Personally, I found getting up and reading was the best way to stop the insomnia panic, and, as the HRT removed my night sweats, that made all of it easier.

If you know, you know

HRT has helped me hugely but, before I even started taking the hormones, I had been able to define what was wrong with me after seeing Dr Newson, and that's where my comeback started. A grain of confidence had been restored. I wasn't going mad, I wasn't alone and I did not have a mystery terminal illness. I was just a woman at the end of her fertile years grappling with her body's response to that. I was more in control of it all again and I wasn't a failure. I didn't have to cope with the shame that I had lost all my coping skills. The relief was overwhelming. Once you feel physically better you can start to work out what else is going on, because you're in a more reasonable place to think.

There are many books out there (all listed at the back, see page 236) that can help you define what you are going through, and online there are gazillions of useful fact sheets and questionnaires you can take to your GP to help you get support too.

The terminology can also play a significant role in all this. I don't see perimenopause and menopause as an illness; it is a hormone deficiency. I'm just replacing the hormones I have lost. I am treating a problem with a solution, as I would diabetes. Joining the dots of older women's healthcare in this way is beginning to become more important – it will, after all, save the NHS money in the long term. We all want to be healthier for longer, so I am urging you not to get side-tracked by the nonsensical 'natural' versus 'not natural' debate. Body identical HRT, which the NHS guidelines recommend, is made from plant extract; it is natural (bio-identical HRT, however, is not; it is the form of unregulated HRT sometimes prescribed by costly private hormone clinics as lozenges). Taking body identical HRT is not about going down a 'less natural' route; you cannot replace fluctuating or declining hormones in a more 'natural' way.

Right now more research is being carried out on the female brain and how the changes to it during menopause can affect our future health, not least because women have a greater risk of developing Alzheimer's – the biggest killer of women – than men. We have 10 times as many oestrogen receptors in our brains as men, according to neuroscientist Dr Lisa Mosconi, which is at the root of many of the physical and mental symptoms we encounter. Oestrogen is what the scientists call 'the master regulator' and without it we may notice a significant dive in the quality of our mental and physical health (hence the anxiety and depression some of us encounter for the first time in midlife). This drop in oestrogen also seems to be linked to our increased risk of Alzheimer's.

Many medical professionals are now starting to view

perimenopause and menopause as a long-term hormone deficiency, rather than supporting the narrative that we should all just put up with the symptoms without replacing those hormones or adapting our lives to alleviate them.

So now we know. Time is marching on and we're all starting to be better informed about what's happening to us physically and mentally. The taboo is being lifted. And this is all good, but I can't help thinking this new medical knowledge, while useful, may also help portray this stage of life as a worrying and frightening time for women. The problem is that attitudes to older women in our white, Western society are still mostly negative; we live in a culture where ageing is seen as a negative thing, where women are not valued unless they are younger or fertile, so the medicalisation of the menopause can add to the confusion and distress – one more thing to feel shame about in our ageist society.

Medical experts tell us there are many lifestyle changes – exercise and nutrition in particular – that can alleviate the symptoms ahead of time, which many of them are now writing about. For example, a blood test showed that I was extremely lacking in iron – common in perimenopause – and because I now knew what was happening to me I was able to adapt my life to support the new needs of my body. Out went the exhausting cardio exercise and in came yoga and weight training to support my bones. Dr Annice Mukherjee's book *The Complete Guide to the Menopause* is useful for those who do not take HRT and therefore want to concentrate on lifestyle changes instead. Having gone through breast-cancer treatment herself, she lays out many alternative avenues of exploration.

If GPs were to lean towards a more socially prescriptive model of patient care, in which they were to advise women in their late thirties about what changes to expect in the years to come and how to plan for them, this could be helpful for the next generation.

I spoke to Dr Vikram Sinai Talaulikar, a menopause and reproductive medicine specialist, about this after a tweet he posted on the idea of a positive midlife transition prompted a heated thread of responses.

'Many cultures value all their elder people more than we do in our Western cultures. Communities look after them well,' he told me. 'I see many women from Asian, Middle Eastern and Afro-Caribbean or African heritage who don't want medical intervention. While on the one hand this subject is not talked about in their communities, the attitude for them is about positive change with age. Often there is a lot more respect in these communities for women as they mature.'

'This release from having periods, this end of contraception and what is consequently sexual liberation is seen as a good thing,' he went on. 'In some Indian communities, women are invited into powerful decision-making roles at this age alongside the men.

'Of course, equality of roles is the ideal all the way through life, but when the message is that older, post-menopausal women are more powerful, more revered, valued and respected, then younger women in those places look forward to this age, whereas here we often dread it because we place so much value on our youthfulness.'

When Vikram tweeted about this idea of menopause being a positive experience, many women felt that it implied that their symptoms were again not being taken seriously (as we know, many of these symptoms are debilitating), but I welcomed the idea that in many cultures older women are so much more respected than they are in our own. That this stage of life is seen as positive for older women. The concept of 'the elder' – the notion that we transition into a wiser place after we have gone through this physical change in life – is one that I think we should fully embrace.

Awareness is, of course, much needed because a more positive language around this stage of life should be available for everyone. Not all women need medical intervention, but those who don't should not deny the experience of others who do – that's unkind. As Vikram pointed out to me, we should really be talking to women in their late thirties about the perimenopause and menopause and counselling them so they can make any necessary lifestyle changes in advance and perhaps have more regular health MoTs to identify any underlying conditions that might not have been addressed as thoroughly as they should.

'There are a lot of lifestyle changes or mindset changes we can make as we head to 40, which would ensure a happier, healthier old age,' he said. This can mean altering our diet and the kind of exercise we do, as well as taking steps to reduce stress. But we're still so frightened of talking about women ageing, about women's health generally, that we haven't joined the dots on this.

I feel we must make more of the positives that come with no periods, the end of childbearing and a release for many from monthly hormone hell. Often a powerful, healthy, energetic rebirth follows the perimenopausal years – a 'second spring', as Vikram calls it – and yet little is spoken of it.

'No one is talking about the menopause as much as they should, but I see a lot more negativity towards it among my Caucasian patients than in other communities where it is not viewed as a bad thing.

'I wish that message would reach more women, because while it is wonderful to get all this medical information out for women, it would also be wonderful to impart a sense of liberation and joy too for women.'

Vikram says almost all the white midlife women he sees seek medical intervention as a first line of response to their symptoms, while women from other heritages will see medical intervention as a last resort.

'It's interesting to see this different approach, and of course,' he adds, 'many cultures simply won't talk about these aspects of women's health at all, which is not helpful, but I would like to see a more balanced conversation for women about how we manage perimenopause and menopause – a conversation that is more positive and less worrying for women.'

Many of the women I chat to in midlife tell me they feel a huge surge of energy post menopause. Most have made lifestyle changes that have reduced stress. One midlife listener to the podcast stopped me randomly at a book launch to tell me she had taken up weightlifting at 50 to get healthier as she aged: 'It gave me back my libido, my confidence and my sleep. I have had many lovers since I started with the weights!' she remarked. She was not taking HRT but had realised exercise and sleep quality were crucial to happiness.

Every voice is relevant in the championing of women's health, and until now none of them has been heard, so bear with us while we make the noise needed to keep many women alive longer, or living a good life, with or without the support of HRT. Changing this negative perspective of older women in Western culture is starting to happen, and it will continue as long as we all remain open-minded and inclusive of each other.

All the rage

I feel at this point that I should tackle the Tony Soprano-like rage that floods through the veins of midlife women. It's a surprising symptom of getting older, but feeling overwhelmed with everything life throws at you after 40 will irritate you at the very least, or, as in my case, drive you to apoplectic fury. It's an 'outsized' rage, too big for any of us to handle, and we don't wear it well. It feels like being Basil Fawlty furiously explaining the difference between a rat and a hamster to hapless waiter Manuel all day, every day.

In the 2022 sci-fi horror film *Everything Everywhere All at Once*, the simmering fury of the constantly overwhelmed main character, Evelyn, perfectly sums up this rage to me. The film also features one of the best movie villains created: Jobu Tupaki: 'An omniversal being with unimaginable power, an agent of pure chaos with no real motives or desires,' according to the movie, which is how I think many of us feel at midlife when the rage hits.

I've often transformed into something out of *The Shining* in the face of a toaster that won't play ball. I have been close to savaging a supermarket self-checkout the moment it tells me assistance is needed. My teenage son once asked a Tesco employee to step back: 'Leave her alone, man, she's raging,' he said.

Sometimes the rage was so all-encompassing I would have joined any march for any cause just to stomp angrily around in a crowd of other angry people. Perimenopausal women should hire themselves out to boost the activist numbers!

Once I started HRT and my sleep had improved, my fiery rage reduced but did not entirely disappear (as my husband would say, I was still TAT – tetchy all the time!). I don't know what would have happened if I had had to go on without the right form of medical support. I think my marriage might have ended, because I was so irrational and cross with everyone, and my libido was non-existent too. At the very least I believe I would have stepped out of my job for a sabbatical. More importantly, though, it would have done irreparable damage to my relationships with my teenage children. You need lakes of parental patience during their adolescence, and I would not have had that without HRT and the knowledge of what was happening to my body.

So what is going on inside us to cause this blind fury? Dr Louise Newson explained to me that the neurological reason for the rage is part and parcel of the extreme mood swings perimenopausal women may encounter. She said that oestrogen helps regulate our serotonin, a neurotransmitter that carries signals between the nerve cells of the brain. This serotonin is the 'feel-good' chemical that keeps you happy, but when your hormones fluctuate the regulation stops, so no oestrogen, no feel-good feelings; instead, you may get the opposite. If you combine this with lack of sleep (sleep is a regulator of mood chemicals too) and the consistent low-level stress of being utterly overwhelmed, you can see why your brain may pick fury as your default emotion.

Because, yes, neuroscience and endocrinology aside, being overwhelmed is likely to be one of the sources of your extra-mean reds. The building sensation of stress-induced burnout is not just a physical problem, it's an emotional one. The glass has to over-flow at some point. Holding it all in constantly, as Gen X has been taught to do (women aren't supposed to be older or angry in plain sight), is exhausting, and inevitably it will come out. The incessant task of ticking things off the work to-do list and the home to-do list simultaneously can't end well, can it?

Even in the most equal of relationships or the most heavily resourced and financially supported homes, most women still do the bulk of the thinking, the organisational planning, the emotional heavy lifting and generally running the family's daily needs. The have-it-all generation (more on that later) seem to have realised later in life that the immense pressure of this emotional labour notches up the mental temperature close to boiling point. And let's not forget that women of this generation have been told most of their lives that showing anger is not 'ladylike' – it's viewed very dimly in women generally, so we have learned to hold it in. I stopped holding it in when I hit the wobbly phase. I mean, I couldn't have held it in if I had tried – it was like wrestling a giant, furious bear to the ground: impossible. I wonder if a snake feels this huge, furious sense of restlessness just before it sheds its skin . . .

I also wonder if, as they look back in midlife, Gen-X women have also started to re-evaluate their experiences during the '80s and '90s in a culture that was hard on women. You've only got to watch things like the original *Top Gun* with anyone under 25 to see how consistently women were demeaned and diminished. My 11-year-old asked why women weren't allowed to fly planes in those days (1986) and if they all had to wear high heels to work at military airbases? It was probably relentlessly rage-inducing and may have made us subconsciously cross all the time, and that's before #MeToo came along, triggering memories from that time that many of us then had to come to terms with.

So if you are wondering where your own rage has come from, know that it's the result of years of manic activity and pent-up fury crossed with the neurological effects of a lack of oestrogen – a combination that would make a powerful weapon of mass destruction if you could harness it efficiently. But also remember that rage may be a sign of psychological pain; as the US priest and philosopher Richard Rohr once said: 'If we do not transform our pain, we will most assuredly transmit it.' And of course it may also show in the body – fury is not good for the nervous system.

Now for the good news!

Thankfully times are changing and women in midlife are increasingly being seen and heard; we're making a noise and getting more support than before. For my podcast co-host Trish and me, gathering all this midlife knowledge has felt a little like discovering the whereabouts of the holy grail of women's health. We're able to spot women in perimenopause after just a few minutes of making small talk with them! Occasionally women come up to us when we are out and about and tell us we've saved their marriage or their career with our podcast, or that they have finally worked out how to access HRT, which has made life bearable again. They were less cross than they had ever been, and this is wonderful for us to hear.

Midlife women may be invisible to most of society, but for us they loom large. In a changing room by the side of a freezing lake on one of my many early-morning swim jaunts, I listened to a woman discussing leaving her job at a bank. She told her friend forlornly that she just didn't think she could cope anymore because she couldn't sleep and she kept forgetting everything. She was not herself; she just felt awful and rage-filled all the time.

'How old are you?' I asked (a lifetime of being a journalist means you do this without thinking sometimes). 'Forty-six,' she replied. 'Then you are perimenopausal,' I said. I told her to listen to Dr Louise Newson on our podcast and to get herself to her GP, but to be ready to go to another GP if the first one offered antidepressants. I gave her a link to the NHS website and the Balance app, developed by Dr Newson, which is the most thorough source of advice and medical support on the subject in my opinion (see page 234 for download details). Trish and I are like a roving perimenopause ambulance service.

And as the show became more and more popular and the number of downloads hit the millions, we heard similar story after similar story. It's amazing, we'd comment after each celebrity podcast interview, that so and so has never talked about all this before. All these women who feel the same at this stage of their lives, women from so many different backgrounds, all wondering what's going on inside their hearts and minds. What a coincidence!

And then the lightbulb went on. We realised why all our Gen-X guests had never talked about the rainbow of feelings they were being hit with in midlife before: because no one had ever asked them.

101 Things Only Midlife Women Know: Brain-fog Bloopers*

~ You forget to put eggs in the pan to boil. When you look into the pan your first thought is, 'The eggs have dissolved.'

~ You accidentally check out someone else's shopping trolley but don't realise until you're unpacking it at home.

~ You take the three sausages you got out of the fridge to defrost upstairs to your bedroom.

~ There's half a cucumber in the airing cupboard and last night you took the dog bowl up to bed with you instead of a glass of water.

~ You've got someone else's glasses on your head.

~ You remove your eye make-up with your HRT gel after a rare night out.

~ When you see your 17-year-old sellotaping her door key to her ankle to avoid losing it (again) you consider doing it with your keys too.

~ You take the shoes that didn't fit you back to the shop and give the assistant an empty box, because you are wearing the shoes.

~ You go back to the shop to collect the phone you left at the till but when you get there you buy a magazine instead.

~ You address your friend's birthday card to her pet.

~ One morning, post-shower, you brush your underarms with your toothbrush.

~ You load the washing machine with clean, unfolded washing and forget to put it on.

~ You get into the shower wearing your bra and pants.

~ You try to open the supermarket doors with your car alarm key.

* (These have all happened.)

3

Sloth Sunday

It's Sunday. One of my two teenage daughters is walking round our kitchen like the bored long-term inmate of an open prison. Dragging her feet slowly, she is taking the tea bag carelessly out of the cup and dripping it across the floor to the bin in the manner of a giant sloth. 'I am so bored here I could sleep myself to death,' she says to no one in particular.

Is that an option for me? I wonder. Would that be simpler, easier all round right now at this middle bit of life – an endless sleep? Would that rid me of today's confusing feeling of joylessness and loss, this out-of-character blanket of meh that seems to have descended? Would I have to tell anyone I was doing it, though? That feels bothersome, too much of an effort. Is it something I have to dress for? What would be my last meal? How comfy is the bed? I need a harder mattress than most. But who would do the laundry, change the loo rolls or remember to get stuff out of the freezer? No one else knows the Netflix password.

My WhatsApp begins to ping with Sunday updates from the other midlife females in my world. Women I like very much. These WhatsApp conversations are a pithy sitcom crossed with an intense docudrama. 'And just like that . . . they all went mad' type of thing. Our WhatsApp has morphed into an unofficial catalogue of the Unmet Needs of Gen-X women; it is a chronicle of amusing and not so amusing unravellings.

Some threads unfold like an Adele album from her future, the one with 40 or 50 on the front. Divorces, reunions, dating dilemmas, sex-toy mishaps, dysfunctional family shenanigans, drugs at dinner parties, intimate injuries, domestic injuries (mostly involving that slicing devil, the mandoline), dark humour on the diagnosis of terminal illnesses ('But she has been teetotal for 10 years, how can she have cancer?'), unacceptable levity in the face of the seriousness of dying relationships – all human life is here minus pregnancies and births. Some tales are as dramatic as storylines from *Big Little Lies* or *Desperate Housewives*. I kid you not, bruh (as my three teens would say).

The new unpredictability of these women, my women, astounds me. So much is going on now most of us are in our forties and fifties that it is hard to keep up. All the big existential questions seem to come up on the chat and are at risk of being tackled by a group of women uniquely unqualified, and too emotionally unstable (or hot, as in boiling hot), to answer them. But we mostly seem to be asking versions of: 'What is wrong with me?' or 'what's the point of me?'

Life has unexpectedly strayed into unfamiliar territory, and it has made some of us doubt things, question things. We all feel a loss and a bit lost at the same time.

This pause between Act One and Act Two of life – the 'mental pause', as one of us dubs it, because most of us feel 'mental' – is a series of contradictions. It is lonely, but also liberating; tingly too, as if we are on the brink of something giddy and powerful. But some of us seem to have come unstuck here, which is a surprise. We don't know who we are or where we belong. We're not complaining (well, some of us are) or moaning (don't like to make a fuss); we're perplexed (and occasionally depressed). We are clinging on. We want the fun back, that feeling of carefree fearlessness and hope in our lives again. We want stability, not this shifting quicksand. Or do we? It's hard to conclude anything with concrete certainty, frankly.

We have an unexpected, unfolding sense of loss of one thing or another: the loss of youth, of status for some, of fertility, of our now-grown-up children leaving home, of our parents, of our status at home and at work, of memory, of relevance, of our looks, of our libidos, of our waistlines and obviously almost all our collagen. At times we feel diminished by this ageing process, invisible even. And overwhelmed – it's an unexpectedly large amount of loss to grapple with all at the same time and it seems to be throwing us off-course.

We have to tackle larger than-life questions pertaining to chaotic out-of-this-world scenarios that we didn't envisage we'd encounter: divorces, affairs, terminal illnesses, teenage shenanigans, redundancies. Expectations have not been met for some. We're not quite who we want to be or the woman we were. Not that we're even sure we want to be her anymore anyway.

People we love have left us: some of them have died, some of them are dying, some have walked away. It's all too much, we're too much, and we can't cope with the unpredictability of not knowing what might happen next. In this place there is constant change, and it is discombobulating.

In dangerous times in dangerous seas, they tell you to keep your eyes on the horizon to remind you all will be well, the storm will blow over, but for us the waves are too big to see our horizon. The storm is all-encompassing; the waves may wash us away.

And it's not that we're resisting growing up or getting older. I, for one, have surrendered to that. I am not putting up a fight or seeking a to-do list for my second-act epiphany, and I certainly don't want any slogan tees with inspirational quotes on them about getting older, or daft nicknames for my tribe. We just want answers to why our dials are slightly off. We feel unprepared and we want to know what comes next. We are the sticky-back-plastic *Blue Peter* generation – some of us have Brownie badges (not me) – and if we knew what to expect, we'd be better prepared. But we can't see many role models around us who've found the answer.

My CEO friend Gina has been unexpectedly orphaned at 56. She has become unmoored from her dock after the death of her parents and has begun clearing everything out of the house with such manic energy that I am afraid for the dog. Will he go on Facebook Marketplace too? It's as if she wants to clear her previous life away to stop remembering, but you can't put grief on eBay.

Mary, once a high-powered city financier, has taken up needlepoint – 'It calms me,' she says – and started shopping for clothes in garden centres instead of her normal upmarket retailers. 'I swear to God, it's the softest wool you ever felt,' she messages one morning about a new cardigan. She's a completely different person. Another high-flying friend has gone to the US to 'study' climate change on a whim. Inexplicable.

The message threads also fill with lengthy discussions on our mothers-in-law's hip surgeries or the dreaded 'fall' they've had. There's a divorce looming, a divorce happening and a secret affair unfolding on WhatsApp. Women are kissing women. There's serious illness, lumps being discovered, therapy beginning and the unbearable sadness of an attempted teenage suicide. There's self-harming daughters, adolescents struggling with eating disorders, mums whose eating disorders have 'come back', husbands who've come unstuck, a gender transition for one son, redundancies (expected and unexpected), career reboots, sabbaticals, depression, antidepressants, diets and manic exercise fads.

There is also the emergence of the entertaining epidemic of midlife hypochondria among the sexes. The midlife men in our homes now seem to suffer from all manner of exotic ailments and this peppers the chat with humour that deserves a 10-part Netflix series.

'All he does is go to the doctor,' Caroline types. 'Everything requires medical attention, from a nosebleed to indigestion, while I am just getting on with it. And I've got a torn anus,' she adds, referring to the ongoing surgery required after having two baby girls two years apart, each weighing over 10lbs at birth, more than a decade ago. Our own mystery ailments take up space too: is it rosacea or some rare tropical disease? Google is inconclusive. Breast cysts are drained, moles removed.

This runs alongside the elderly-parent storyline, which is as laugh-out-loud funny as it is worrying. A few of our octogenarians revert to being teenagers, it seems, as they age: at times duplicitous and irreverent, sneaky and tricky, eluding us with their unexpected escapades, taking off on trips when they've been told by medical experts to stay in bed. A friend had to park her own car across her elderly dad's drive to stop him speeding off on unauthorised dates in his ancient Volvo.

A few midlife husbands or partners have morphed into strange beasts to cope with too. My friend Asmah laments the weight of emotional labour she deals with at home, despite her husband now working from the kitchen they (she) are refurbishing. 'He is like the fourth child,' she adds. 'I have to ask him to repeat everything to me out loud after I have told him what's happening, or he deliberately forgets and the windows go in upside down. I have to do everything.'

Another husband has run off to Spain with a colleague 12 years his junior – he's a new dad again at 52 and desperately trying to find a way out of that responsibility, as he did with the previous ones. We call him the 'man-child' and wish all manner of suffering on him in support of the woman he left after 30 years.

CEO Sally spends her days making everyone redundant, she messages me. 'They make me do it because I am the grown-up,' she says. I would not call Sally grown up; that is not my experience of this podium-dancing raver who once woke up in a window box clutching a Big Mac. The woman who often walked over Westminster Bridge to work at 7 a.m. from a subterranean nightclub under the arches at Vauxhall. This is the woman she still thinks she is, by the way; it's just that her colleagues cannot see this side of her because they haven't known her 30 years.

Mira is 54 and single and has adopted a one-year-old after an intense six-year process. She hasn't had time for the menopause or perimenopause. Another friend has developed midlife allergies that are getting out of control. 'It's inexplicable,' she types. 'I can't even look at a full-sized banana without coming out in hives. The little ones are OK, though.' The allergies complement her sudden-onset acne at the age of 48.

'All I need now is a lovebite and a perm and I will look exactly like I did as a 17-year-old,' she types.

Two of my friends tell me they have been diagnosed with ADHD. 'It's sort of a surprise,' one types, 'but it explains a lot,' before adding, 'actually it doesn't really explain anything. I am not sure what any of it means anymore.' Me neither, I reply.

Some of us are grappling with the misbehaviour of our adolescents, the shame of some of the things they do, the shame of how we react. How could we have raised such dreadful humans? we ask each other. How could we be such dreadful parents? Did we let them down?

At one point our ever-increasing collective brain fog feels like an epidemic. 'We can't all have Alzheimer's,' I typed one morning on the way to work, wondering if it was something in the water in London. How can we all forget everything all of the time? Is memory loss more contagious than chicken pox?

Occasionally we move on from our ailments to the ailment to end all ailments: death – usually the inexplicable sudden deaths of people with six degrees of separation from us. The friend of a friend whose boyfriend had back pain and then died of cancer six weeks later; the ex-colleague who suddenly has the brain tumour we all fear we have due to the memory bloopers; the record-company PR we all love who doesn't wake up next to his wife one morning. We talk of death until one of us breaks up the chat with a reminder that this is why we don't ring our parents so often; they're 'Radio Obituary', playing Top Trumps with those they've outlived. The ending of endings seems so unfair, so illogical.

And just like that . . . my career is over

Our WhatsApp messages are peppered with a new indecisiveness (where did that come from?), a decline in confidence, a gradual loss of the things or feelings that 'light you up inside', as one friend puts it. We also often feel an unwanted sense of irrelevance. We feel a little invisible, gliding through our days without being remarked on anymore, being taken for granted by family members and colleagues. A midlife mum tells me her forgetfulness has become so bad her teenage daughter regards her as even more of a moron than she did before.

'She's on my case all the time,' the mum says on Facebook.

‘WHAT'S WRONG WITH ME?’

‘I made her a cup of tea this morning and it was too milky. "You must do better, Samantha," she reprimanded me.’

‘Must do better’ is the phrase rolling around in my head. I feel like a student who has suddenly dropped all her grades and been asked to take a year out. All I know is that my new identity, my Act Two life, has to be forged with purpose and optimism. It has to be consciously decided on, not fallen into.

As teenagers we rolled into life without really thinking it through – maybe we set an identity by accident and our life then flowed round that personality – but surely this new life stage is the chance to choose who we want to be, rather than getting swept along as we maybe did in our hope-filled youth, that former life with an abundance of time in it? Maybe my new identity will be like Doctor Who regenerating . . .

On the WhatsApp we wonder if we can go into an old people's home together, the home that seemed a million years off, until yesterday when the invite to the opening metaphorically arrived.

‘We'll advertise for staff for our old people's home on my new fantasy website, Frenchtotty.com,’ Caroline types. ‘It's just pictures of handsome French men who fix things for you,’ she explains. ‘They can bring us our G&T enemas.’

‘You can't say that anymore,’ we all reply. ‘"Enemas" isn't rude,’ she says. We should cancel ourselves, we conclude; our humour is tainted by childhoods spent watching Carry On . . . films and Are You Being Served? These were the days when Anthea from The Generation Game was sold to us as a female role model, and being a Bond Girl as an acceptable career choice. No wonder we're so confused.

Some of us are still in denial about the ageing process, even while we note that so much time has passed that Chardonnay has made a comeback – our teens tell us about it as if it is a new drink. They have never heard of Bridget Jones.

48

I begin to look purposefully back over my shoulder into the past with a new sense of clarity, but this is like opening a box of fireworks that promptly go off all over the place. You often see things differently with your midlife specs of retrospect. Some of the experiences that shaped you, helped define your identity, unveil new thinking. They make uncomfortable viewing some-times, these memories. I wrestle with unexpected doubts around them, questioning past decisions in the way only a woman who frequently says 'I have absolutely no regrets' can. Ridiculous me.

Time seems to be going faster but I know instinctively I should be taking things more slowly, because, as we all agree via our chats, perhaps the decisions we make now really do matter. If only we weren't going mad, we'd be able to make more sense of it all. We feel the pressure to make all the right choices at this crucial middle stage, whatever 'right' means. Our mortality is breathing down our necks and people keep sending us cards with that Mary Oliver quote on them asking what you are going to do with this 'one . . . precious life' . . .

Back to the Sunday afternoon in our kitchen with the tea-dripping sloth. On this day in my early fifties, I am just feeling down for no reason, very much wondering what the point of it all is. I don't have a hangover, the usual precursor to this Sunday feeling.

I am taking my HRT now so it's not hormones, not physical. I've enthusiastically taken up wild swimming, I've listened to all the wellness podcasts and even started one of my own. I am doing all the right things. I have ticked the mind and body checklist of make-you-feel-better coping strategies for women getting older, and yet I still feel like I don't belong here, in this space and time. It is strange.

I don't have anything to complain about, but I react very differently to stress these days; it is debilitating for me in a way it wasn't before. Before the pause, in life's first act, I revelled in stress. I could listen to the TV and have a conversation at the same time. Or reverse park with the radio on. I had three jobs and four children at one point. At this point, I am busy editing a weekly magazine for the *Sunday Times*, writing a weekly column, recording a weekly podcast, writing a parenting book, maintaining an active social-media profile, much to everyone's annoyance ('Mum, you're using Instagram wrong,' is my son's favourite phrase), checking in on ageing parents, home-schooling a 10-year-old in a pandemic and co-parenting three teenagers and our Welsh terrier who barks at everything, even leaves falling from trees. So much change all at one time – change you don't envisage in the run-up to midlife. Maybe all of that is the cause of my unease. Then, in the middle of it all, my 30-year career editing magazines comes to an end.

4

Are You Familiar with My Work?

In my study there is a framed fortieth birthday card to me from Madonna. A picture of me interviewing Oprah and Reese Witherspoon live on stage hangs beside it. There's a handwritten thank-you note from Chanel's Karl Lagerfeld after I persuaded him to design a Comic Relief T-shirt for *ELLE* (the Chanel surfboard he gave me for my fortieth lords it over our sofa in the lounge). A pair of white birthday boxing gloves signed by Emma Watson sits beside a mocked-up magazine cover of me and my midlife crush Dwayne 'the Rock' Johnson, who sent me a video wishing me a happy fiftieth.

On the floor of this tiny room there's a big box stuffed with career memorabilia, glamorous and historic debris from the worlds I have floated through over three decades: film, fashion, art, politics. In one picture on the wall I am sitting with all the female members of Tony Blair's cabinet at Number 10 for my *Cosmo* editor's letter. On a postcard actor Jeff Bridges thanks me for using his pictures from a film set in *The Times Saturday* magazine. The Eurythmics' Dave Stewart apologises in a note to me at *Marie Claire*, where I was features editor, for messing up the recording of his Demi Moore interview, and reminds me 'he isn't a trained journalist'. Me neither really, Dave, me neither, yet several journalism and magazine awards also sit on my study's top shelf. All this memorabilia has remained largely invisible to me over the years but, looking at it through my retrospective specs, the Aviators of time, it is as if it has all happened to someone else. 'Who was that woman?' I wonder, as I navigate career grief in my new jobless, office-less, colleague-free life after exiting my final role editing the *Sunday Times Style* magazine.

Maybe that's why I have had to put an all-persons bulletin out on my lost identity in my early fifties. I've gone from these globe-trotting adventures to post-redundancy 'sadmin', as we call it, in 2020: sorting new email addresses, mastering Google Drive, wandering from the study to the kitchen in search of biscuits to have with my tea as I embrace this new career as a writer and podcaster.

I feel like I have survived a particularly ridiculous performance by an immersive theatre company, like the time I mistakenly agreed to see the You Me Bum Bum Train stage show in a derelict four-storey warehouse. This was a troupe of hundreds of volunteer actors who took audience members one by one through increasingly weird scenarios over a two-hour time frame. I went from being crowd-surfed at a rave, to being trapped in the trunk of a car, to a plastic surgeon's operating theatre, to a vet's surgery where a dog was being put down, to presenting a cooking show, to the back of a truck simulating the police discovery of hidden refugees and, by bizarre coincidence, the imaginary HQ of Chanel in Paris. It was the most disturbing thing, and none of it made any sense – rather like looking at my study wall of life stories now or into that box of career memorabilia. What was *that* all about?

Who exactly was I now after menopause, after motherhood, after all my years at the helm of something that felt important and influential to me, at the top of a career I had built? And how had I landed in all those rooms across the world?

I left home and my Cornish comprehensive school at 16, moving from a small bungalow on an estate at the edge of Bodmin Moor to a shared student house in Streatham to work on the *Wimbledon News*. I was incredibly lonely when I first came to London, before I gradually melted into the life I dreamed of then. I felt that loneliness nipping at my heels again after I left full-time work in the summer of 2020. I was wandering around a metaphorical new place, a place where I didn't know how to fit in yet. At the same time the eldest of my four was about to leave home, and the pandemic was changing all our lives.

In those first moments out of my job I felt I was being pulled downstream in a river of uncertainty, still clinging to the sturdy log of my editing career for comfort, but I realised instinctively that I had to do the hardest thing of all and let go. I couldn't panic or grab on to the next thing that came along.

A month or so after I left the *Sunday Times* I remember standing in the shower watching the bubbles bounce off the floor in a trance as flashbacks of my life engulfed me and a new perspective formed around them. I started to view Act One differently.

The story I had told myself was that starting my career so young was a brilliant move, tying my identity to it so tightly, so early, as many of us did if we didn't get the chance to go on to further education. I was blind to any other opinion on this decision. I had also assumed a full-time job would be my forever path. And, of course, it was comforting over the years that people seemed continually impressed by my background. Other people's approval gave me the glow of achievement. This positive story of a self-made, working-class, comprehensive-school-educated woman seemed to surprise everyone. People's eyes would pop when I answered 'none' to the question of which uni I went to. When I worked in newspapers (*The Times* and *Sunday Times* especially) I was mostly in rooms where everyone answered Oxbridge to that question.

I obviously didn't have the foresight to predict what it would mean decades later. I had tethered myself so strongly to the job that we were intertwined like ivy wound around ancient trees, all knotted up. It supported me. Until my family came along, it was the most important thing I had. How would my editing career and I separate in the least painful way possible all these years later?

It was June 2020 when I received the phone call many print editors were getting after decades in the business. I was part of a trend, but, unlike the drama of perimenopause, I was much more prepared for this.

The well-paid highfliers had to go to save cash. My part of the media industry didn't need so many of us anymore. As the conversion to digital took over, print media was seeing a drop in advertising revenue and the audience was heading elsewhere – to podcasters, social-media influencers and online content creators.

I'd been told how the future would look on the magazine I was editing, and it didn't appeal to me. I'd enjoyed the best of times and wanted to swerve what I felt would be the worst of times for me. I could see that the easiest way to save money was for me to be the saving. It made sense, and besides, I had a side-hustle: I was a podcaster, social-media influencer and creator of online content. So while I was 'out', I was also 'in'.

Even so, nothing prepares you for saying goodbye to the stability of the thing you have been for most of your adult life. I had to leave the team and the office, to swiftly and suddenly exit a career that had started with a typewriter in a tiny room above a Liskeard newsagent on the *Cornish Times* and had ended with page impressions on the *Sunday Times* at the top of a building in London overlooking the Shard.

Newspapers and magazines were the love of my life and suddenly I had to say goodbye to being part of that world every day. And the pandemic meant I would not be able to observe any of the neurologically soothing rituals you normally go through with such a big transition, such a final ending. No leaving do, no Colin the Caterpillar cake. Instead, a card and present biked round with a box of my belongings. I was catapulted out of my comfort zone into an unusual place (as many of us were anyway during lockdown). It was all very weird.

I wasn't jobless. I had the increasingly successful podcast and two books to deliver, but I was in a world where I didn't belong, with people who weren't my tribe. Every time I met someone new I had to explain who I was, when previously my career had been so easily defined it came before me when I entered a room. I'd spent years working and socialising with the same set of people and most of their lives were carrying on in the same way while mine was changing irrevocably. I was bewildered by it all and looking for the imaginary guidebook on how someone bounces back. And while I knew that no one was indispensable in my industry, I had hoped I was the exception to that rule. I think everyone does, don't they?

I felt a bit sorry for myself, even though part of me was excited and optimistic about the 'what next?' aspect of it all. I just had to endure this 'before then' bit first, find my new path, didn't I? But how?

Now I no longer had that day job, now two of my four children had left home, now I wasn't Lorraine Candy from the *Wimbledon News*, from *The Times*, the *Mirror*, the *Sun*, the *Sunday Times*, the *Daily Mail*, no longer the editor-in-chief at

ELLE or *Cosmopolitan*, what was the point of me? (As my teenage daughters often asked.) If your head is always tilted in one direction, it's tricky to balance and find stillness when the thing you're tilted towards suddenly disappears, isn't it? As I searched for purpose in my new future (you may want to read this in the manner of Carrie's voiceover from early episodes of *Sex and the City*), I looked for clues from the past.

In 2015 I'd worked with an executive career coach, Alex Villars, who specialises in big change. I had turned the *ELLE* office into a digitally engaged hot desk to modernise the glossy mag world. I sat with the team, moving places daily. As you can imagine, this caused uproar. Change was hard, so to make it all less painful for everyone, jovial Alex came to coach me through it as the team leader.

When I called Alex to chat about this latest big change in my life – the equivalent of not just having no desk, but no longer being in the building – he and I discussed burnout, which he said he had witnessed often, due to the majority of his clients being high-ranking men and women in midlife.

I like Alex – he views things with a Buddhist overtone, while at the same time acknowledging that his clients have to keep the cash rolling in. I was after clues as to my new working identity, which would be useful to my working life now. How would I deal with making less money and being less important?

'You had little empathy with your team as they struggled to accept change,' he recalled of my time at *ELLE*, 'because you had little empathy for yourself. Big change can only come when you have empathy for yourself. You were very much like many members of your team whose identity was "I am what I do"; your attitude was just "get on with it no matter how painful it is". You were quite hard on yourself and I recognised your mindset as perhaps a more male [one] in a female-dominated environment. You had hardened yourself in order to be taken seriously in that world,' he said.

'It is a particularly Generation-X trait actually, and I see it often in women of the Thatcher generation. The "I am fine and I can cope" mentality. I think the next generation of women [millennials] have a softer way of working for themselves and for others; this is not about it being a more feminine way but a more human way,' he concludes.

In a long conversation, Alex and I went on to look at how women like me – I guess you'd call them highfliers, which doesn't make them more important or more skilled, just part of that particular tribe – cope when it all changes. One of the notable characteristics of this tribe, he said, is an addiction, and in my case it was probably an extreme addiction to being manically busy. This trait doesn't suit midlife when, as Alex tells me, leaders start to conclude that the currency of time is more important than the currency of money or status. How best to spend that time therefore becomes of the utmost importance, because of the sudden appearance of our mortality.

Finding busyness, of course, is a default way to avoid stepping into the void of transition between your old life and your new one. But at some point the 'doing' has to stop and the feeling has to start. It took me two years after the end of my office job to soften and slow down, to resist the lure of this addictive busyness. It's still a work in progress and every now and again my podcast co-host Trish will step in and quiz me on my manic activity. It's such a default setting of mine that I have to actively press the stop button. I had always thought being constantly busy was a good thing, and of course at times it was, but the relentlessness of it was not healthy.

The untelling of our life stories as we age and our transition into new places is a fascinating revelation in midlife. Looking back made me realise that holding on to this certainty of purpose, this ambition, had left me unable to settle, to be in the moment, to just see what happened next, which is a much-needed midlife skill that I, and many of my contemporaries, were missing.

This change to our way of being is 'a process', and I've learned that it's not wise to rush immediately into something similar to what you were doing before after such a big change at your midpoint. Don't immediately grab what you are offered or take up something manically time-consuming to distract you from the uncomfortable feelings that this retrospective on life may throw up. You might have to say cheerio to something you loved – that will be hard, and you'll miss it deeply, so give yourself time to adjust. I cherished my days editing magazines and I relished the manic mornings at home before heading to the office, so I had a bit of grieving to do in saying goodbye to that stage of life before I could move forward.

I have also learned that you should perhaps be questioning everything that has happened in your past, exploring it (celebrating it too), and not finding some way of numbing all the feelings this new stage of life will trigger: with booze, extreme exercise, any kind of drama or excessive 'doing'. Take a moment to sit purposefully with your memories: remember your successes, re-evaluate your failures, learn from all the things you have experienced. Doing this helps you think about tomorrow in a new way. It sets you free from expectations as well – yours and those of others around you; it's a letting-go. We can learn many surprising things about ourselves when we look back on events through midlife's more mature eyes. I think at this point in life right now some of us may secretly long for 'softer times' – squidgy marshmallow days, as I saw them. When the walls around us aren't so hard and stiff as they were in the past. Our outlook evolves and becomes less rigid, our behaviour more fluid. Maybe we realise the panic will pass in the middle stage of life (it does) and that we're just being put on hold for a little bit, which is perhaps a good thing.

When my job first ended, I worried about how I would validate myself externally after stepping out of such a clearly defined role. If someone asked me what I did for a living when we were out, my husband would visibly flinch. He was worried I would find this new lack of identity mortifying and that my sea-witch midlife rage would surface. I think he feared I would bite someone (he's a non-confrontational type of human).

Who was I if I wasn't all those busy, needed women I had once been? If I didn't have that status? But here's the thing: along with all those anxieties, I also felt hugely relieved, like the weight of a massive cloak had been lifted off my shoulders. I was surprised by this feeling because, ultimately, I am a bit of a show-off (when I did that famous 16 personalities test it revealed I was 85 per cent extrovert). I was proud of my career as an editor, yet I felt oddly cleansed after my initial gloom. It was most disconcerting. There appeared to be little grieving for the status. It was more for the people.

Three years later and I still feel surprisingly relieved not to be a boss anymore, not to be representing an organisation of any sort, just being in charge of myself. Maybe mine is an unusual reaction, and certainly I was grateful for the privilege of having earned enough money not to feel immediately worried or desperate for me or the family financially.

And I had the financial cushion of our podcast, *Postcards from Midlife*, and the creative nourishment of book-writing to lean on, which helped for sure. And maybe I had subconsciously created those in anticipation of this turn of events? Who knows? People seemed to imply I'd been smart to do so, but really it was accidental, the by-product of being manically busy all the time. Which is ironic.

I still had to earn money, but not as much as before, because as the dynamic of our family of six was changing, my responsibilities were lessening financially. It was all oddly good timing.

What bothered me, though, was the lack of defined structure in my day and the loss of my colleagues. I was lonely at times. I had no sense of belonging, and that was the biggest bereavement I had to come to terms with: the loss of regular office life, of a mini work family around me. No one to nurture, no bright-eyed young people with all that optimistic energy. I missed that, and the uncertainty of what I would do next was where the fear lay for me; the lack of clear definition on the road ahead destabilised me. I felt as if I had not been in control of this change, which I didn't like. I didn't take the loss of my job personally, and I don't think it affected my confidence as much as other things did, though the loss of my earning power was something I would have to come to terms with, but it left me at the beginning of something for the second time in my life. What that something was I didn't know exactly.

I felt guilty for any negative feelings I had because my life was OK. The leaving wasn't a shock, I was lucky to be where I was and to have achieved my ambitions, I wasn't dissatisfied with my family, my marriage, my world, so what had I got to feel discombobulated about? I had my HRT, too, so physically I was coping. And I knew so many women who'd hit midlife and found themselves in a crisis of fulfilment: nothing they'd dreamed of had come true and time was running out, so unfortunately disappointment reigned for them during this complex time. I was grateful not to be in that place, and to be presenting a podcast where I interviewed women about this again and again was undoubtedly helpful. I was also so grateful to be healthy, a thought that had rarely entered my mind until midlife. I'd taken my health for granted up until then.

I was absorbing advice and experiences like a sponge from all the women I interviewed, with gratitude. The midlife army was there for me, which is why I wanted to share all this with you, to make you feel less alone if you are going through a huge transition too.

Dropping the ball

At first everyone at home tiptoed around me, apart from my two eldest daughters, who did what most much-loved teenagers do when someone else is in a time of crisis: they worked out how they could most benefit from it! As I grappled with existential questions about the end of my career as an editor, they kept making use of my extra time at home that summer by sending me on errands. I was always off to get them something from Boots and they persistently asked me to make them breakfast at 2 p.m. on Wednesday afternoons when they were home for the holidays. I was like Baldrick to their Blackadder that summer; it was 'yes, m'lord' every five minutes.

The teens seemed oblivious to me losing my job; their only concern was that I was writing a book on parenting adolescents. 'What would man know about that?' they would ask dismissively in teenage slang, before high-fiving each other for their wit and making the 'L' for 'loser' sign on their foreheads.

When copies of my book first arrived in the house one of them commented that it 'smelled nice' and nothing more was said. I was, as all parents are on the surface, irrelevant to them (it is the way with teens as their brains develop, so I didn't take it personally or blame them).

When they dismissed me like this, which I knew they would do whether I had a job or not, it unwittingly hit a bit of a raw nerve, because at this stage my relevance was in question in every way, wasn't it?

I had only ever been at home and away from the office for such a long period once before in my life, when I was on gardening leave between jobs, and then I'd written a lengthy piece about how I wasn't built to be at home.

To avoid overthinking things, I started to listen to Radio 2 and would occasionally watch *Escape to the Country* or *Real Housewives of Beverly Hills* between writing and recording, while the rest of the world was at their office desks. My schedule was no longer 9 to 5; I would write before sunrise to avoid the busy house, and the podcast was recorded in the middle of the day. My work duties were now ad hoc. Which I felt oddly guilty about. I had to define my own diary and fit in all the domestic duties that needed to be done: school pick-ups, breakfast for the kids, shopping, laundry (being home also meant we no longer needed part-time help with childcare). I was in a completely different kind of daily role.

At times it felt a little like one of my maternity leaves but without the agonisingly painful nipples. All of it made me itchy for the predictable regularity of the glamorous office life I had had before. Anna Wintour (editor-in-chief of American *Vogue* and a magazine contemporary) wasn't watching *A Place in the Sun* of an afternoon, was she? I would ponder as I chatted to the dog settled on my lap. Anna wasn't wiping Super Noodle grease off the kitchen worktop after the teens' 2 a.m. cook-ups, was she? She wasn't accidentally filling out the wrong month in her Google diary and turning up to Teams meetings when she was supposed to be on Zoom or actually in the room.

At first I was subconsciously thinking, 'When this is all over . . . when it all goes back to normal . . .' – an illogical mindset because it would only be 'over' when I was dead, wouldn't it? Change is continuous at all ages, but I don't think you realise this fully until you hit midlife.

A wave of exhaustion swept over me in about month nine, after my first book had been published. It was a success, and the podcast was still growing, proving to be an excellent distraction from the 'what next?' question that everyone kept asking me. But I was overwhelmed. I had kept the diary so busy that it had floored me.

I'd occasionally feel so 'unusual' I'd have an afternoon bath (in the week – who does such a thing?). And then I'd be so tired I'd take a nap. One afternoon I was woken from my nap by my 10-year-old after I'd forgotten to pick her up from school round the corner on the one day she'd asked me to. I felt ashamed. I was so used to remembering every tiny detail of these things; it was out of character for me to forget this whopper of a must-do.

My husband kept checking up on me as if I was a nervous new pupil starting at a different school. In truth, I'd come a little undone and was being unnecessarily manic in all the confusion of how to fill my days without the rigid structure of an actual job. I was defaulting to what I knew. Like a lab rat. I think he was worried I'd join a cult or start volunteering. Instead, I just 'did too much'. Which, as we have discussed, is the perfect distraction from feeling too much.

Indeed, there are some things that you should *not* do during this time: get your new passport picture taken is one (I look quite unhinged in mine); finally engage with your immediate neighbours after a lifetime of just nodding hello (I was moments from joining the Guinea Pig Alliance on the Nextdoor app at one point); watch bleak films like *Nomadland* on your own at the cinema in the middle of the day to make you feel less bleak about your moments of bleakness; buy clothes online made by tiny boutiques in small European countries to support the woman who runs it and because the embroidery reminds you of something (you will never wear them); grow your hair under the mistaken impression that you now have time for the 'in-between phase'; start a list of 'projects' you always said you'd get done but haven't (they didn't get done for a reason: they aren't worth doing); announce that you will spend more time with your husband to your husband – he doesn't know who you are now any more than you do, poor bloke. And his own midlife crisis doesn't welcome change. Plus, he has probably already been through a bit of a ruckus with you during the perimenopause – his hairline can't handle any more.

Switching states takes more time than you might imagine, so, if you're in the middle of it right now, be patient with yourself and do nothing for a bit (you'd be surprised how many people alongside you are also slowing down. I was amazed at the number of non-retirement-age women out and about during the day when I stopped working in an office).

Stop and think – after all, this is perhaps that midlife crisis everyone talks about. Do a bit of investigation and research on what made you you to help you figure out who you might be now. Look back with purpose. Do less, not more. Release your-self from your emotional responsibilities and leave spaces in your day for nothing if you can. Delegate stuff, drop the ball, leave stuff undone. Saying 'No, thank you' is also a new habit to embrace.

People kept ringing me to ask if I was OK in those first few months after my job ended, but because I was so busy still saying yes to everything, I didn't notice the extra layer of concern in their voices. I wasn't open to new experiences; I wasn't curious enough. I really wish I'd been brave enough to sit with the discomfort of all those feelings I was distracting myself from at an earlier stage, to take a proper break, because I would have reached a happier, less stressful place a lot more quickly. I think I needed boredom and silence, and some 'alonement' too – a term coined by writer Francesca Specter to mean fulfilling, quality time spent on your own. I needed to train my body and brain not to expect this busyness, to let a different skill bubble up, to feel a little compassion for myself and be more vulnerable. I was striving for a reinvention, which is an exhausting goal in midlife, when perhaps evolution was something better to aim for. And I felt guilty that this turn of events wasn't more gruelling for me. I felt guilty about the privilege of my circumstances, as if my situation didn't rank highly enough on the chart of midlife trauma. I had no sense of being able to enjoy the moments initially, opting instead to just do more.

Many women around me of my age were also either stepping out of big jobs or being pushed, and at times my departure felt more muted, less dramatic, than most because I had other hills to climb, even if I couldn't be sure if they were the right ones yet. Of course, I realise mine is a tale of ease in many ways. I was lucky to have full-time work, but a slower mindset would have proved useful, offered me a better way to handle this ending emotionally, especially during a pandemic just as my eldest left home.

I know many women have to step back into jobs after redundancies, that many have to earn money to support their families, but small changes in mindset that take you to a softer, less critical, less manic place will ease the transition, even if you have no choice about work. According to career coach Alex when I chatted to him, this slowing-down mentally has to be a purposeful decision. He suggested a re-evaluation of what you need, a taking stock of circumstances.

One of our podcast guests during this time was a business highflier, who had taken what she called a teenage year out. Michelle, who left a council house in Birmingham to come to London and build a staggeringly successful career, told me she would get up late during her adolescent experiment. She didn't bother to brush her hair, she watched telly for hours, used a different mug for every cup of coffee, bought some giant trainers and routinely left them in the hall for everyone else to trip over. She refused to eat fruit and played with the dog in the garden for hours. She talked endlessly to her friends on the phone, sat in Starbucks and walked around her neighbourhood at the speed of a sloth. It was a revelatory period, one which resulted in her recently launching a new business, which has since become a global success (infuriating, I know!), but she maintains that taking the time out to do nothing saved her soul and her physical health after her previous 30 years at the top of her business.

'I'd had a teenage son,' she explains, 'so I just copied what he'd done one summer.' Maybe we all have a version of this, even if it is just a daily one?

I am, of course, aware that we don't all have the luxury of being able to take time out, but if you are moving out of a big role in this stage of life, just be careful not to step into exactly the same role again. And if you are feeling this itchy loss of identity but have to keep working, ask yourself if you can make your days kinder to yourself. Can you review the way you work, and your mindset around it?

Many women I've spoken to were chasing reinventions, some of which would have been exhausting. They told me they wanted their 'ambition' back, but would that be good for them? Maybe abandoning ambition was OK. Can you mentally unravel yourself and your identity from your job, your mothering, your caring – whichever role you have been tied to for so long? What would that feel like?

This midpoint in life is an important time of evolution whatever your circumstances, so consider how you can make your daily life easier to help you cope with these big feelings – feelings you should not avoid. The overriding piece of advice I got from many who'd been through it was to take the time, feel the feelings – good and bad – and keep a mental list of your small daily wins. Note the things you could do that would allow you to slow down and acknowledge where you are. There is a lot at stake for Gen-X women and this default do-it-all mantra of ours doesn't serve us well.

I hate to go all Oprah Winfrey on you, but this really is a time of soft introspection, of caring for yourself more thoroughly and not feeling guilty about that. I wrote a list of non-negotiables at one point during my post-redundancy wobbles (such an out-of-character thing to do), a list of things that had to happen in the day to keep me grounded and less panicky. Stabilisers. A hot coffee on my own first thing with the kitchen window open, a swim once a week, cuddles with my youngest at bedtime, a glass of water first thing. These became the small daily habits that helped regulate my moods. I knew if I could purposefully do one or more of those things in a day, life would be OK, calmer even. Sure, it's touchy-feely wellness waffle, but you know what? It works.

5

Generation Burnout . . . Are We There Yet?

The wind is so strong our crisps fly out of the bag and back into our faces. We're sitting on a wooden bench in the local park in our jogging gear during one of the lockdowns. Mischel has brought the 'luxury snacks', as we refer to them; Mira has brought three cans of gin & tonic from M&S. We couldn't carry too much – we're on a jog, after all. It's Friday at 6 p.m. and it is cold and grey. We did the run but now we're on a bench trying to combine a drink with a jog – a 'drog'. We're staying fit, fighting off the middle-age spread; this is the debit–credit lifestyle of the Gen-X woman.

At this point in lockdown my friends and I are still unable to meet in our homes and we've grown bored of sitting in my front garden wrapped in blankets. 'You're like those women camping at Greenham Common when you do that,' one of my teens points out, using an uncharacteristically accurate '80s reference.

So now we do this 'drog' thing and endure the cold, windy bench together because endurance is our middle name. Gen-X women are good at endurance, like Antarctic explorers plodding forward in a blizzard of confusion, dragging a giant sled of responsibilities behind us. We're the explorers – the Scotts, the Amundsens (I wish I could use the names of famous female explorers here, but it looks like the patriarchy stopped them leaving home). Endurance is linked to men, but it's women who endure the most in my opinion; we're the copers, a band of self-sufficient realists. Which is perhaps why we're so shocked when we hit this tricky middle patch; we struggle to endure it, or finally find we can endure no more.

As a generation we don't like to moan about our 'failure' to cope with it, or whinge – it upsets everyone around us, so we try to muddle through. But this thing is harder than reaching the South Pole; the mental and physical load is too much to drag without help, especially at it appears to catch most of us by surprise.

We'd like to push on successfully but we're too busy patiently FaceTiming the foreheads of our elderly parents to discuss their prescriptions, googling 'dry vagina normal?' and counting the minutes of good sleep we've had this year on one hand.

We are confused as to why we're not coping, not enduring, and we're drawn to each other in the confusion of figuring out what comes next. Who are we as our careers end or change, as mothering comes to a halt (almost), as our finances wobble, as our marriages go into meltdown, as our health throws us a curve ball or the work of grieving creeps up on us?

Who are we when society side-lines us, makes fun of us with hot-mess stereotypes on greeting cards and more or less excludes us from stage and screen at around the age of 45? Who are we as our earning power diminishes because we step out of jobs to raise families who have now left us? No wonder we feel worn out and left out.

In a thread on our *Postcards from Midlife* Facebook page, women who are strangers to each other gather to discuss their midlife transitions and share their nagging sense of loss of identity. I notice that the most frequently used words are 'burnt out' and 'overwhelmed'.

Panic has set in for the over-forties because time is running out. Burnout – as career coach Alex Villars pointed out in the previous chapter – is a specific ailment of Gen X, who are experiencing not just career overload, but also life overload. Expectation overload, duty overload. As Ada Calhoun wrote in her book *Why We Can't Sleep: Women's New Midlife Crisis*, for us, middle age can feel exhausting.

Ada began researching the book after 'the worst of summers', she says – the midlife summer when she felt alone and broken but then discovered she wasn't when she interviewed 2,000 other American midlifers. Their stories made her sad and angry, but they also gave her hope.

'For some of us this time is a legitimate crisis,' she told me on the podcast. 'Women [of this generation] are doing so much; it is not possible to go through all that and not feel a sense of panic, which we feel ashamed about because we are supposed to be able to cope, to have it all.

'It would be revolutionary for this generation of woman to say, "What if I can't do it? What if I can fail?" We've internalised all the messages we had growing up that we had all these opportunities so we must do everything and be perfect and have a career and a family; it is hard to let go of that internalised ideal, especially if we don't have it by this stage of life.'

She added: 'It feels like we need permission to talk to friends about this, but once we do there is a sense of feeling less alone. Then we feel seen.'

If you combine the Gen-X work ethic with our family responsibilities and perimenopause (which we have only just found out about), it is easy to see why we specifically find this stage of life so hard. We don't have the toolkit for coping with it, despite our endurance mindset. Those who have gone before us didn't have the same responsibilities.

So it's no wonder we all feel like we do. It is not because we are failing; it's because we have not been armed with all the information. After all, no one told us about self-care until around 2010 – until then, we still believed that things like yoga were an expensive waste of time, despite what Oprah and Goldie Hawn have been telling us for four decades!

You are not alone

Many midlife women (and men) reach this point and feel the four Ds: despair, defeat, disappointment and dissatisfaction. Expectations have not been met, life may not feel how it was supposed to feel, physically, emotionally, practically and financially. It seems unfair and entirely understandable that some women have come up for air after decades of working, or parenting, or caring for people, and are furious that they're miserable after so much endurance. They're cantankerously unfulfilled. Our midlife rage may start with fluctuating hormones, but it also comes from that Gen-X female feeling of having to do everything, 'allofthetime'.

And many have landed in what may also feel like a period of contradictions; we're older and wiser but at first we are oddly less confident than we thought we'd be. We may care less what people think but we're too overwhelmed to make the most of that liberation. It's a topsy-turvy time of opposites after all that enduring. I felt a bit of a failure for not being able to manage my life as well, for not being able to deal with stress. For forgetting which side of the road to drive on.

But I also noticed that some women are suddenly grappling with the strange possibility of contentment instead of achievement or ambition – a new concept for us manic Gen-Xers; less martyrish, but trickier to get right. Could not coping be a choice, or asking for help, or delegating and saying no? Or just giving up on it all for a quiet life? And why do we feel so guilty about doing that?

A nurse on our private Facebook group wrote: 'Has anyone experienced a career crisis in their late forties? I'm unsure whether I'm burnt out, frustrated by my new job in the same field that hasn't quite met my expectations, or ready for a complete change of direction.'

A long and helpful thread built up around this post. The thread was an impressive army of midlife women gathering around one of their own in turmoil; it was a 'no woman left behind' mindset. Their comments were inspiring – powerful evidence that we're not all slowly going crazy, and that if society wasn't listening to us then we could at least listen to each other.

Many who responded said they had stopped sleepwalking in their forties and had experienced a form of awakening. The 'no fucks left to give' era, as it has become widely known, perhaps offered the chance to endure less and enjoy more.

I should point out, of course, that midlife isn't always a tale of struggling to keep your head above water, in case you were worried this book is turning into a bleak 'meno noir'. Life after this 'mental pause' can be liberating and joyous, as we shall find out. But a great many of our Facebook midlifers posted about being ambushed by an out-of-the-blue feeling of failure. In Natasha Carthew's memoir *Undercurrent* she recalls the Cornish phrase 'nothing is left behind in an autumnal tide', which struck a chord with me. This is what I felt many women were describing in this period of their lives: everything having been dragged out by a force beyond their control, the great autumn tide of life, leaving them feeling empty.

'I've achieved nothing,' one lady wrote. 'I'm 50, divorced and will never afford my own home now.' Again, the midlife tribe massed around her, telling similar stories and looking for the small wins of this game. 'Me neither,' one woman replied, 'but I have two lovely sons and a new boyfriend; he's poor too!'

As I read these posts about careers, domestic life and endurance, about coping with divorce, the death of parents and the loss of jobs, reinventions, new loves and lives, it felt as if I was looking into these women's windows at twilight, watching them plotting and planning for a new dawn in the midst of their home life, many quietly laying the foundations for something different, or just a new attitude.

It's not always about attempting an exhausting process of reinvention, which is a narrative we often read about when trying to overcome the hump of midlife. That narrative I feel has strongly stereoptypically male overtones – an achievement mantra. It seems to me that the process of acceptance and continuing evolution is more helpful than dramatic reinventions and new starts. Or maybe it is about adapting our mindsets to not let our own harsh thoughts, judgements and criticisms derail us when things begin to fall apart or change – trying not to turn our thoughts in on ourselves, whatever the situation we're in, whatever we begin to observe about ourselves at this stage.

Many of these women had encountered imposter syndrome too, especially those who'd gone back into the workforce after becoming mums. Their loss of career confidence as their identities wobbled posed extra challenges. One told me there is nothing more demoralising than being interviewed by a man half your age on Zoom, especially if you can't work out how to turn the filters on to look less tired.

'I just looked at him and thought, "He'll never understand how bringing up three kids, including a set of twins, with no help is like being an air-traffic controller at Heathrow in

August; he just thinks I have been making cup-cakes and wiping butts,'" she concluded.

The word that comes up again and again as I unpick the issues around career identity is 'threshold'; women of the endurance generation seem to meet a threshold they have to cross in order to redefine or find themselves at this age. To know themselves better rather than reinvent themselves. These thresholds can be in their existing job or the gateway into a very different kind of life (such as, of course, stepping over the threshold out of motherhood, but more on that later).

I don't think we have been given the tools to navigate the crossing of these thresholds, or been given them clearly enough, or even heard other women talk about dealing with the menopause in this way until the past three years, when the conversations began to unfold publicly, with high-profile women sharing their experiences out loud. Instead, we've had to face making big decisions at a time of life when we are grappling with so much else.

One thing is for sure, though: no thresholds are going to be crossed unless we 'get off our arses and cross them', as career coach Rachel Schofield told me when I rang her to find out how we can find a less fearful way to approach our confidence crisis at this age.

'I think we often get to this point in our lives as women where you become the last priority in a long list of things to do. Changing things to benefit you seems to be the least of everyone's worries, which is unfair,' she said.

'What we seem to hit is confusion around who we are. First, we need to start believing in ourselves again before we make any concrete decisions on what [comes] next at home or work. This is a process that takes time, and before you get anywhere you must sit in a void . . . and it is uncomfortable for a while.

'This is not a simple rebirth,' Rachel tells me. 'That's not what is going on. I encourage women to trust the process, the journey, and to find moments of revelation on the way. You are not just going from A to B; that's how it may feel, but actually you don't know the end destination yet. Many women are really surprised by where they end up at this stage of life and what they eventually choose to change or do.'

One the first things I learned was that the busyness of my previous life, the relentless hum of my hectic schedule, left no space to wonder if this was actually what I wanted to be doing for the foreseeable future – or even the next few hours.

When I first left my role at the *Sunday Times* I assumed I'd focus on finding a new job, but it slowly dawned on me that I didn't want to be employed again. I didn't chase or accept the stuff that first came into my inbox, which surprised me. Financially I wasn't under immediate pressure to do this, though that time would come, and we would all as a family have to adapt to having less, but still I doubted myself every time I said no to something permanent on the career front. This lack of ambition was new to me. It made me curious, and, if you're in that place right now, you'll notice that if you stop 'doing', you start thinking (and overthinking sometimes!). And as you do that, all sorts of odd memories pop up. You remember the work highs, for sure, but a showreel of lows may pop into your head too. And these can come from way back. For me, it was as if my brain was trying to finally figure out what had happened now that it had time to file the memories away neatly, rather than shove them messily in a drawer as it focused on what was coming up next.

When one of my former bosses interviewed me for her midlife website she recalled how, when I was in my early twenties, 'we could throw anything at you, no matter how busy you were, and you'd just say yes and do it'. I was proud of that for a few minutes, then I began to wonder if working like that was a good or a bad thing. What effect did it have on me and all those other young Gen-X women, just saying yes and using our endurance to push on through? In those days four weeks of holiday a year was too much to take. Why did I choose to work so hard? Was it ambition or fear? I had nothing to fall back on: no qualifications, no family financial support. It was all down to me. Maybe that was the reason. Even when I married and then started my family I seemed to fall for the exhausting notion of 'having it all', making that my responsibility too.

Sorry, did you mean, 'Do it *all*'?

Bear with me for a moment, because I'd like now to investigate that notion of 'having it all' a little more. It is, as I quoted from Ada Calhoun earlier, at the root of this endurance mindset for Gen-X women. And having worked closely with *Cosmopolitan* founder Helen Gurley Brown, the woman who came up with the phrase in 1982, I have some thoughts on it.

I joined 'the Flamboyance', as I would refer to the group of global editors of *Cosmo* magazine, in the year 2000, when I was made editor-in-chief of British *Cosmopolitan*, aged 31. Getting the editorship was an incredible privilege for a magazine junkie like me. I gave up my job as features editor of *The Times* to go to *Cosmo*. I was offered the chance to become one of *The Times*'s news editors to stop me going, and even though I knew that was an incredible role for someone with no degree, I loved magazines too much to say yes. *Cosmo* would be more fun.

A year later I found myself in the Bahamas with all the other *Cosmo* editors from across the globe. After a day of 'conferencing', we stood in the blistering heat watching Helen Gurley Brown hurtling down a perilously high water slide in a skimpy red swimsuit like a character from the film *The Incredibles*. I feared for Helen, fragile and bird-like as she was, but she emerged perky at the other end of the slide – which had passed through a dining room and an aquarium. A butler wrapped her in a fluffy robe and she slipped back to her penthouse suite (to coiffure her hair into its familiar back-combed bouffant style). She was almost 80.

I had never met a woman like Helen before. She had shaped a long-lasting cultural narrative, which had defined my generation for good and bad: the idea that we could aspire to have it all – work, love, family and financial independence.

The mistake we made, I see in retrospect, is that we also took that to mean DO IT ALL. We saw it as an instruction. Doh! We didn't want to drop the baton for the women behind us after we'd been given such a new opportunity. It was less a blessing and more a burden.

The problem was, society wasn't set up for us to 'have it all': it had been constructed by men who didn't envisage us standing alongside them at work or them alongside us at home. And so, in trying to have it all, we changed the schedule, didn't we? We gave birth later, which meant some of us still had a young family in our later forties and early fifties, the time when we'd be higher up in our careers, and more financially and personally independent. We stayed in education longer. All the timings were out.

School pick-up schedules didn't serve us well, and flexible and remote working was unheard of, but we couldn't be in two places at once, so we constantly felt we had to choose one or the other. Society didn't celebrate the notion of blending work and family – we even called it the 'struggle to juggle', as men stepped aside, watching us instead of supporting us. As the years went by we also realised that those men who did immerse themselves physically in home life, with or without children, still weren't doing any of the thinking and planning around domesticity; they were still opting out of the emotional labour of it all. Many suffered, too, from what has been labelled 'weaponised incompetence', where they would wait for instructions on how to help, because most still saw it as 'helping'. In other words, it was *our duty*, but they were learning how to help out as a favour to us.

When I once quizzed a male boss of mine, who also had four children, about how he managed to balance his career and domestic life, he looked perplexed at the question: 'My wife does all that,' he replied, failing to see the irony of who he was talking to.

Having it all was impossible, and it was unforgivable that sometimes we tried to make it look easy so other women didn't get frightened off from giving it a go. Successful women told us to lean into it and dream big, but they didn't offer us ways of doing that, so we struggled with the set-up. Having it all was a ruinous phrase; it was potentially liberating, but the misunderstandings around the messaging and the lack of male support made it ridiculously unrealistic. It did not propel us forward out of servitude (something only wars and states of emergency had done before) as we'd hoped. It placed a hideous pressure upon us.

If the world had been built as a more equal, better balanced place (constructed by women, even) then 'having it all' would have meant something else. Instead, it was and is a mess. I am aware that I am talking mainly about my own demographic here, but there are a lot of us around and the effect rippled across all of society.

It just didn't work out for us as Helen, the most successful glossy magazine editor in history, saw it. She had launched *Cosmo* in the US in 1965, when she was in her midlife, aged 45, turning a dull literary title into a go-getting, feminist (sort of) monthly based on this having-it-all premise. The idea clearly appealed to women because *Cosmo* became the bestselling women's magazine in the world, dominating newsstands in every country where it was launched.

During the time I edited the UK edition Helen had a stranglehold over *Cosmo* globally and I adored her spirit. I admired this tiny, pencil-thin powerhouse so much I could ignore her obsession with dieting and dating, her bizarre habit of valuing women for their looks, which all seemed counterintuitive given her other messages. Instead, I focused on her rallying cry for abortion rights and female financial independence.

Helen had defied what she called her 'poverty-stricken hillbilly' background and had made it right to the top. She demanded that doors opened for her at the White House, on Wall Street, on Park Avenue and in all the fashion capitals of the world. She once surprised us at another conference by introducing a secret guest: she'd secured us an audience with Woody Allen (who at the time was a notorious recluse, known only for his films).

I watched her in action with awe. This woman had lived more lives than I could imagine, her identity so firmly formed by her extraordinary career – one she didn't step out of until the day she died in 2012, when the *New York Times* wrote, 'She died in Manhattan aged 90 – though some parts were considerably younger.'

So in conclusion, my friends, I think this notion of trying to 'have it all' is the reason many of us feel so burnt out in midlife, and why it is peculiar to our generation. If you're wondering why you can't endure all the things all the time anymore, given everything else that may be going on in your life, then take into account this have-it-all mindset and whether it has played a conscious or subconscious part in your life.

My attempt at having it all came to an end when I exited *Style* magazine. I left the building with a bruised ego. I was in the doldrums (which sounds like a place from Radio 4's shipping forecast), because I think we all like to hope our final exit from the building only happens if the building is dramatically on fire behind us.

I had now lost the structure and the routine, as well as the approving nods of colleagues accepting my years of experience. I was, after all, the boss, and everyone agrees with the boss. At work I was an MVP (most valuable player); at home, where I now was for most of the hours of my new life, I didn't get that respect. The teen girls saw me as a cross between Bart Simpson and the pensioner in the car adverts called Morag. In fact, my son still calls me Morag. (I rather like it now.) I was an NPC – a non-playable character in video-game parlance – an irrelevance, just wallpaper. My 18-year-old would often ask me what I was doing as she passed me in the kitchen. When I told her I was working (writing and podcasting) she would look perplexed. 'But you haven't got a job,' she would say. 'Shouldn't you be at Zumba or something?'

As the months passed I began to relish the control I had over my own time; it felt like a privilege. I had never had it before. There was no sense of time being my own during those having-it-all years. I know this state was easier for me as I had a degree of financial freedom – always precious when you don't come from that kind of background – but I still felt both liberated and useless at the same time. It was confusing.

'This midlife reckoning is like doing a giant jigsaw,' career coach Rachel Schofield told me. 'You get the edges done first and that's your first big win, then it starts to gradually come together, and you find you are enjoying the process rather than focusing on the end picture . . . It's about being patient and happy to own all the bits of you, including, for some, the sudden lack of ambition, or a loss of confidence. It's a challenge, and you are not just fighting with how society values you . . . you've got that internal battle going on too.

'And it isn't that we don't want to change, it is that we don't want that uncertain bit which comes before change. It's the bit where we have to redefine ourselves and explain ourselves, which we . . . fear people won't like or accept, especially when we start to say no to things . . . But it can feel freeing when you liberate yourself from the need to transmit an explanation of yourself to everyone.'

Rachel also told me the instruction she gives to the midlife women she coaches: that we reframe the idea of an 'old me' and 'new me' and focus instead on the evolution of the 'one me'. 'Then you feel like you have agency in the process,' she explained. '[It] isn't "happening to you". You can try and find some power and control [in] what you expect the outcome to be as you evolve.

'Part of the reason we lose our confidence is, we begin to feel we don't really know ourselves and therefore how do we present ourselves to others? This can look like a lack of confidence when at times it is just you taking time and thinking about what you're going through. Society doesn't buy into us taking time out to do that.

'If you stepped away from your job for motherhood, you may have had quite a solitary few years and now you are looking at reconnecting in new ways, taking a new perspective on life. I think women are also always under a microscope; if we are not at work, society is wondering what we are doing all day. Men don't get this. So many of us are tied up in doing things, sorting things, which we don't shout about out loud. We are not doing a specific job so we stay quiet about what we are doing to our own detriment or because it can be dismissed as not being valuable sometimes. This all plays into our sense of self as we age.'

So midlife is an identity minefield: whether we've worked full-time while raising a family, not had a family, only had a family. All of it requires huge shots of endurance and a commitment to an overwhelming purpose, and then, without warning, it all changes. The roles fall away or transform dramatically, and suddenly your age comes before you into a room.

This comes with a sense of loss. Our purpose is less clear. Our mind and body are changing in ways we didn't expect. We're off-script and tempted to press the panic button. But women have gone here before us, and experts have studied this pause between life stages. What they have learned can guide and reassure us as we sit in this space, this new void. It's a place we have to go to before anything else can happen.

101 Melancholy Midlife Thoughts That Will Wake You Up in the Night

~ 'Death maths'. You had never heard of that phrase until it started to make you sit bolt upright in the dark. Death maths is the time you have left versus the things you want to do. It is always a smaller number of days, months, years than you thought/hoped.

~ Wondering who will die first. If you're in a relationship, especially a long-term one, this thought had never occurred to you before, but now it is a daily intrusion, which comes with variations on how the first person to go will go.

~ The last big row with your teenager when you called them something awful, then they went out for the night and now you don't know if they are alive and if their last thought was how much they hate you. This is basically 'was I a good mum?' played out via many different night-time scenarios. It will still wake you months after it happened.

~ The times you told your elderly, possibly now-deceased, parents you were too busy to call, pop over, help with the garden, answer the question that started with 'You remember your biology teacher . . .'

~ The faces of those you have lost. These haunt you and you sometimes think you have seen these people in the crowd during the day. The younger versions of them, the ones you knew back in the day.

~ That mole on your back is definitely cancer because cancer is coming for you. During the day this is illogical; during a perimenopausal night sweat it is the only thing that is certain in life for you now.

~ Things you have lost, such as precious jewellery that a lover, partner, parent, deceased friend gave you. You have no idea where it is. Occasionally you will get up in the night and start looking for it.

~ When the dog will die. You've taken the dog for granted, but the dog is the glue of family life. Will you have to take the dog (or maybe cat, though they seem to worry everyone less) to the vet to be put down? How will you and everyone you are related to cope with a dead family dog, taking with him or her all those memories? Have you got enough time left for another dog?

6

Something Unexpected in the Bagging Area . . . or Welcome to the Void

By this point you may be mistakenly thinking that midlife means you will end up face down in a puddle of doom, living your life to the lyrics of the Carpenters' 'Rainy Days and Mondays'. Perhaps you imagine that the only way to answer the question 'what's wrong with me?' is to do something dramatic: ditch your family to walk a 600-mile coastal path in your flip-flops or abandon your career to scale Kilimanjaro in a bikini.

You don't have to do anything as exhausting as that. What you do have to do is step into a new place that I'm calling 'the void' (better names are available, I just haven't thought of one yet). This is where you pause to sort yourself out.

I know your first instinct at this age is to say, 'Put my calls on hold, I need to see the manager, because there has been some kind of mistake – I'm only 25.' And when someone in their forties says 'people our age' you instinctively look over your shoulder to see who they might be referring to. But the truth is, you have indeed aged, inexplicable as that sounds and feels.

You're not in a Bobby Ewing-style coma, waiting to wake up and be told that everything is as it was, so you now need to step into the void.

The first thing you should know about the midlife void is that it requires a softening – a more caring attitude to yourself, and to everything in general. The rhythm of life is different here, the pace is slower, and most importantly anything could happen. You'll need a sprinkle of curious optimism just at the time when you seem to have stockpiled furious pessimism.

A reckoning is likely to occur in this void (it did for me), and that may not be pleasant. There will be living losses to overcome as the roles you had before gently, and not so gently, end: the mothering (the empty nest is horrific), the career, the family ties, maybe marriages. There will be the physical loss of loved ones and emotional losses too, not to mention the loss of your youthful looks. All of it will add up and need to be considered in the void, which can often feel so vast it could be seen from space.

You will encounter grief for times past in this space, which benefits from being acknowledged with kindness and gratitude. And there will be lots of 'letting go' or saying goodbye to people, things, places, in the void. And it is, let's be honest here, the beginning of the ultimate ending (yours) – or, let's say in a more upbeat tone, 'the youth of old age'.

How can I best describe the void without sounding as if I am about to pounce on you and persuade you to try meditation, or spout some wellness gobbledygook barefoot like a female Wim Hof? I won't ever do that, I promise, although meditation, like yoga, does work (annoyingly).

Finding the void was quite a revelation for me. It has helped – or rather is helping – me reach a more content and reasonable mindset. Recognising where I was on the road map of life calmed me down, as I began to understand that I wasn't alone in feeling lost from my mid-forties onwards.

If I'd known a trip to this void between Act One and Act Two was coming I'd have felt less of a lunatic watching the clock tick down. If I had known I was going to land here, where the concrete patterns of my past melted into a swirly sea of ever-moving change, I wouldn't have fought so hard to control or cling onto the things that weren't serving me well, things that only made me feel stable because I'd been doing them for so long. Familiarity is a good wall to lean on in uncertain times, but it's not always a beneficial one. Some of my patterns of behaviour were unhelpful and only comforting because I knew how they worked. If I had known all about the looming losses ahead, large or small, I would have been better able to brace myself for them and deal with the grief around them.

This void has been called a midlife crisis forever, but it isn't a crisis at all if you recognise where you are and what is going on. For me, uncovering this space between my old life and my next life was a significant step out of the woods of worry. I felt a little less confused knowing it was perfectly normal to hit this kind of turmoil.

The void, you see, can be a jolly uncomfortable place to be. It involves letting go of long-held behaviours and beliefs, maybe even a future you that you thought you might have, or identities that don't work for you anymore. It involves feeling all the uncomfortable feelings before you move on to what's next, and dealing with some of the more painful stuff in your past that you may have ignored or been deliberately distracting yourself from up until this point.

This 'time between' is about a breaking of patterns. Beware, though, because it is also a place where you can get woefully stuck waiting to figure out what happens next, trapped by negativity instead of looking for the optimistic road ahead of you. And, of course, at the heart of all loss is everyone's least-favourite emotion: grief.

There are so many endings in the void – or the 'fertile' void, as it is often known by mental-health experts, because it is packed with possibility. But the important thing, according to all the therapists, medical experts, older women and thinkers I've chatted to and all the books I've read, is to endure the discomfort and then 'do the work' before moving yourself purposefully forward with a suitcase of new thinking, packed for this next part of the journey. The key is not to rush forward into the same kind of place you've just been, but to figure out who you are, the meaning of you, as your identity and the roles you play change. It's a time of surrender and unexpected revelations.

So how do we tackle this bit? I needed help to explore this void, so I rang the renowned therapist Julia Samuel to chat about it, 18 months or so after I'd left full-time work at the *Sunday Times*. She's an expert on grief, loss and change. A guru of 'the void'.

'The void is the liminal space [N.B. I had to look up the word 'liminal' after this chat: it refers to a transitional point between two states] between your previous self and your next self,' she explained. 'It is where you reconcile with endings and feel the pain of the ending. It's a fertile space; thoughts of "what next?" will come through, some will have seeds of ideas, new ideas – that's the fertile bit – and some germinate, and some don't. You may eventually end up in a completely unexpected place, not the place you thought you would be, an unplanned land.'

Once we find ourselves in the void, many of us may slip into a negative, fearful spiral about what is happening, panicking about what comes next, and what's needed then is a shift in our thinking. As Julia says, 'We sometimes talk about change in a negative way; the language around it isn't helpful, but we can reframe the changes ahead as challenging . . . You can say to yourself that part of thriving in life and growing is to acknowledge[that] difficulties do lie ahead and not to turn that against yourself, not to think you are failing because it is hard.'

We may also try to avoid dealing with the painful bits we encounter in the void. That's a natural response to this part of life as it doesn't have a clearly defined path.

'All life is change,' explains Julia, 'and if you don't adjust and adapt to each phase you may get stuck in them. In midlife it is important to recognise your part in this change process and not to hold on with rigidity to the previous version of yourself. Allow the "not knowing" to come into your life and sit with it for a while. Also, don't conflate feelings with facts during this time. You may feel powerless, but are you? It may not be a factually accurate description of the situation. Feeling things doesn't make them so.'

When I stepped out of my 30-year editing career I threw myself into a million other things to avoid feeling the 'what next?' panic you get in this void. At first I fell into a rabbit hole of depressing thoughts and fears – feelings I would do anything to avoid. If you do that you end up in what Julia calls a state of 'hyper-arousal', which is nowhere near as pleasant as it may sound!

'You can easily get stuck in fourth gear at this stage of life,' Julia explains. 'And if you want to make good decisions about things, you can't be in a terrified or manic state, you can't be scared. You will benefit from establishing regulating behaviours – breathing, exercise, going outside to help balance your emotional system – which make it easier to make the good decisions.'

Listening to Julia – a decade ahead of me on this journey – was a lightbulb moment, a relief. This bit of life was *supposed* to be hard; it wasn't unexpected at all. I wasn't failing to get a grip, I wasn't falling over the edge. All this questioning was normal. There was nothing wrong with me emotionally. I was being hard on myself with these feelings of failure, as so many Gen-X women seem to be.

What crisis?

For those who need more concrete facts, there is science behind the midlife void: it's called the U-shaped happiness curve. In his uplifting book *The Happiness Curve: Why Life Gets Better After Midlife*, Jonathan Rauch explains the research that shows how we all experience a U-shaped dip of emotions around our mid-forties: life becomes less enjoyable, less satisfactory. He calls it a slump rather than a crisis and likens it to adolescence. There's a malaise, a moody midlife time when we may experience the expectations gap: where what we thought would happen has not and others around us seem to be better off in all the ways we see (rightly or wrongly) as valuable.

He says the stress and anxiety of everything that happens in midlife can reduce our optimism bias. And we know an optimistic mindset propels us towards a positive outcome (David Robson's book *The Expectation Effect* tells us this).

Rauch concludes in his book that there is quite a bit of teeth-gnashing before we settle into an appreciation of where we are in life, and this will happen in the liminal space of the void. I can forgive Rauch for totally ignoring the perimenopause (in my opinion men tend to write about themselves) because his book is reassuring on the 'we are all in this together' front and because it shows that we come out of the void happier and more content. Life feels better mentally whatever it physically throws at you because you've felt all the feelings, good and bad. You have survived the discomfort (I want to add 'and no one died', but the likelihood, at this age, is that someone probably did).

Coach and therapist Donna Lancaster, a former social worker, whose work I find most useful, says we should perhaps think of approaching life with a buffalo stance (which couldn't be a more '80s reference if it tried!).

Donna, who wrote *The Bridge: A Nine-step Crossing into Authentic and Wholehearted Living*, explains that during a storm a buffalo won't run for cover like other animals. Instead, it runs into the oncoming chaos, knowing the distress is temporary. It knows the storm is going to catch up with it anyway, so there is no point in running and exacerbating its distress. Likewise, we all have emotional challenges from our past that sit in our soul. According to Donna, facing them in the void is a wise thing to do. You have to go through that process because it will feel better on the other side.

The good news, according to Rauch's research, is that as you age your sense of gratitude and adventure comes back. In his book he cites the scientific surveys around this renewed sense of adventure as further evidence that older people are also more spiritual. The neuroscience shows how our brains change, he says. They minimise feelings of regret, and replace them with a sense of empathy and gratitude. We lose that 'loss of meaning' feeling and, you will be glad to know, we also stop asking 'should I have?' All the 'what if?' conversations peter out as we head to 60 too, he says.

The upward climb on the other side of the U-curve does sound fun. When I talk to women of my generation who are in their early sixties they all refer to this – it's just that you won't believe it until you are there (see Chapter 11). So, 'Chin up, buttercup,' as my grandma used to say.

On a podcast on the WBUR news station, the psychologist Joshua Coleman muses on how normal this midlife feeling is.[9] It is a developmental stage, he says, like teens and their tendency towards risk, and, if we can learn to see these feelings as a normal stage for everyone, then maybe we can stop looking for trauma in it. We'd feel less fearful and confused about where we have landed, and maybe overthink it less too.

Obviously we have to acknowledge that in some cases this emotional dip may be a mental-health issue like depression, but if it is not then perhaps we can just sit it out in the void as we work out what comes next, avoiding any hasty decisions. I have watched many women sidestep their discomfort at this time by distracting themselves with all manner of manic activity or making huge life changes to stave off the prickly feelings. But in doing this you might ignore your instincts; in avoiding vulnerability you may harden yourself too much; in order to cope better, you may not make the most of this thinking time. Instead, a softening is needed.

Looking to external things to make the void feel more comfortable (new relationships, new lives, new careers, new countries, cars, sports) may not be the answer, according to Coleman, because in the void the answer probably lies inside you. Listening more attentively to your own voice, your own instinct, is required here.

Perhaps a realisation that we don't have to be in control of everything anymore is partly where this softening comes in. You can't outrun your own vulnerability when you get to this liminal space, but you can set it free and admit it out loud. The void is a place where perhaps you can stop pretending to be someone else, stop bending around others and what society expects of you, and ask for help. As you explore who you really are after all the parts of your identity have evolved then you can begin to trust yourself more, perhaps even like yourself more.

How to cope in the void

I'll admit, at first, I was a bit of a scaredy cat in the void. My mind was filled with the notion of taking up offers to step back into the same kind of career I had before, yet my heart's instinct was telling me that would most likely be unhealthy for me. I wasn't coping with the discomfort of the void; the slowness of it annoyed me (it still does), my own company was irritating, my new WFH writing and podcasting routine gave me a rash (literally – a stress rash) and I felt a failure because I hadn't found a solution to what came next swiftly enough. I felt like the terrible knot in the middle of a gold chain; some days it felt as if I was just clinging on to my sanity. The atoms of me were pinging off, my identity was disintegrating – I was losing bits of it every day. The tough outer shell of me was exposed and raw and everyone and everything kept painfully poking it. This all sounds like rather self-indulgent overthinking, I realise, but I describe it in detail in case it resonates with you and makes you feel less alone. During this time, I sought out friends of a similar age and asked them how they were feeling. Knowing this experience wasn't peculiar to me was reassuring, so perhaps this helps you too. And I had rather smugly believed that a vision of my new life post the end of my established career, post mothering four small children, would just pop into my head, easy for me to follow.

I am generally an optimistic person and given that I had come so far under my own steam already, I assumed the next step would present itself just as readily, all packaged up and easy to understand. I thought I could order it on Amazon; it was that easy.

Instead, I flailed around in a pool of what I wanted to do, what was financially necessary and what made sense based on what I had done before – and, of course, what I could actually do, having no qualifications and being older than your average new employee. On top of that, I just didn't know who I was anymore or what to do next.

I had to find coping strategies for feeling all these emotions, which included training my gratitude muscle, because apparently I was going to need it, according to everyone I spoke to and everything I read. This annoyed me a lot – how dare Gwyneth's GOOP and its gratitude journaling be on to something – but resistance was futile. I gave in and began to feel happy about the small stuff Buddhist monks wang on about: nature, music, colours, laughter, blah-blah-blah. I began to understand that this whole thing was bigger than all of us.

As I keep reiterating, this book can't be a step-by-step guide to transformation because, as I have discovered, that should not be your midlife goal. Instead, you're after evolution, a hope-filled time of continual change; that's what we need to get used to if we can. This pause in the void feels frustrating without specific rules to follow, but there really aren't any, apart from finding daily coping tricks that make you happier: exercise, better nutrition, regular rest and resets.

I think I first found the void subconsciously when I hit 48. At that point in my life I had begun to feel the first signs of the creeping sadness hanging around me. The kids were 5, 10, 12 and 14. I was still editing ELLE, and had been married for 16 years. During this time, though, my restlessness led me to the water – the cold water of outdoor swimming. This was long before everyone else was talking about it and calling it fancy things like 'wild swimming' (it looks pretty wild the amateurish way I do it, I can tell you). I found that being in cold water seemed to make me feel better about the blues that had suddenly appeared. I was self-medicating for my perimenopause just before I found my HRT.

I can't meditate because it makes me unbelievably angry (make of that what you will), but swimming for long periods of time brought me my first inkling of sitting within the void. And as the years have passed this need to sit with uncomfortable feelings, or indeed to replay tough memories, has grown. It feels daft to say it out loud, but sometimes in doing nothing for a bit we are doing the most important thing. So my advice is to find your equivalent of swimming.

As I gave myself more space in my day I started to notice patterns in the way I behaved – default settings from childhood. I said yes to so much, I was needy for attention all the time and never wanted to be left out. It was all too fast and furious. I tried to do too many things at once, but the times when I stopped and did nothing were the times I began to listen to my mind, to let those seeds of ideas of what next to germinate, as Julia had said. Of course, anyone on the outside could have pointed this out to me before, but I probably wouldn't have listened. I had to see it for myself.

Grappling with this void doesn't mean planning big change; it's more about learning to accept things and shift your mindset around them; feeling with, rather than dealing with, things. We can't always change our circumstances, but maybe we can view them differently, perhaps more positively. Learning to look for stillness helped me cope with the more difficult times, and swimming gave me that stillness; it was a coping strategy. I found that, in learning to cope with the uncomfortable feelings of this transitional midlife space, all uncomfortable feelings became easier to deal with.

Once I had decided not to rush into the next thing and had honed a few coping strategies, I acknowledged that I would need moments when nothing was planned at all, just empty spaces in the diary. This is possible even for those in much more traumatic or busy situations than I was personally, according to psychologists I've spoken to. It's a skill to purposefully find those moments of nothing, to calm the neurological and physical system down. To not feel guilty for not doing or for slowing down. For watching the feelings as they pass through you, rather than instantly reacting to them. Finding moments to take care of yourself a little better and quieten your anxious nervous system, to step out of the fight-or-flight response, which is hard-wired into so many Gen-X women's brains. It requires you to embrace your 'inner sloth', to re-evaluate what makes you feel good physically and mentally. In this place it turns out some of the more annoying wellness memes are actually accurate: self-care is effective even for the most cynical of us (me). This is a time to develop those 'soft skills' we were told were of no use earlier on in life. A gentler approach.

Once you've balanced your hormones and sought the right medical help if you need it, things like drinking less booze, exercising more, moving your body and getting outside in nature are the tweaks that are most effective (there is a list at the back of the book to help you with this – see Chapter 15). Think of adding these good things into your life, and, rather than depriving yourself of other things to make space for them, layer them on top. Maybe I can nudge you to do a little of that even if you still feel the need to stick to your Gen-X to-do list, your achievement goals.

Many women in their mid-forties approach this kind of advice as a challenge, but this more mindful attitude really is helpful. Say no to things, turn off your emails and your phone. Refuse to worry about what other people think, stop comparing yourself to others, stop thinking you must 'endure' everything, stop asking, 'Am I doing it right?' Perhaps pop your guilt about some of your mothering moments aside (you had brilliant moments too), look outwards to your community more, embrace a sense of play or creativity in your daily life, bring back the music. Think about what you want and need but explore your neediness too. Whoever said only you can make you happy was of course right. I often blamed a lot of what I was overthinking or feeling on others around me (i.e. my husband!), but really it was up to me to sort things out or ask for help.

It all sounds so obvious and so annoyingly smug saying it now, and of course I fully acknowledge that I am a white, middle-class professional speaking from a place of privilege, but still, I hope it helps you because this stuff really does work. If you feel this doesn't fit your world or experience of life then please read Donna Lancaster's work: she started her 'softer life' as a Black mum and social worker specialising in child protection but gradually brought the self-care I describe into her life because she knew she couldn't live a healthy existence without it. This mindset change to positivity and optimism is key: there is so much research on this I don't have room to include all of it here, but seek out the science if you can.

Curiosity, adaptability and gratitude are the three things you may need to pack in your suitcase for the trip through the void. And an ability to deal with being alone, though not feeling lonely. It is a bittersweet state of 'becoming' and I would hope it leads to a state of belonging, because the belonging is of course what we may miss the most, for it is our connections to others that are our trump card. That is what will stabilise us, and it should be our priority. Being supported in the company of others is where we will build our happier sense of self.

7

These Women I Like Very Much

Early one sunny but cool summer morning in Cornwall I found myself knocking on the window of a camper van in the car park at Daymer Bay. A beautiful woman in her late forties stepped out, long blonde hair flowing, a faint tan covering her handsome face and a huge, calm smile. I am not one of those people who believes everything happens for a reason, but I do believe in the power of the connections we make, connections that take us over a threshold at exactly the right time. At this stage of life those connections can feel like lifelines; they were nice-to-haves previously, now they are the strongest of ropes to hold onto as you flail around at the end of them.

And perhaps with our eyes fixed on the direction we want to go in, we often find the things we need the most, even if we don't consciously know we need them yet.

At that moment in midlife, I needed Nix Joubert. A free diver, yoga teacher, competitive swimmer, Nix called herself a 'waterwoman'. She was going to teach me to swim faster, to catch up with everyone I often trailed behind in my newfound hobby of open-water swimming.

We spent two hours together that day, but only 20 minutes in the water. Nix had met a lot of people like me before; she knew what to do. The time I spent sitting on the sand with her made me re-evaluate everything, not just my swimming. We didn't get to meet again, even though we'd scheduled in more lessons, but we exchanged many voice notes over the course of the following year. What I learned from Nix wasn't about swimming. She laid out a blanket on the cliff overlooking my favourite beach in the world, the one where I spent my childhood summers, the one beside the church where I got married, and asked me why I wanted to go faster. What did I need from being faster? The question perplexed me at first; she was a swimming teacher for God's sake, why was she asking such a daft question?

'I'm like a sloth,' I said. 'Miles behind everyone. I want to be able to keep up and to swim further and for longer and do bigger challenges. I've got plans.'

She smiled patiently in that annoying way people who meditate do and asked me to consider what it would be like for me if it was OK to be slower. Nix teased me with the idea of tranquillity or being present in the here and now, not striving towards the next thing. And I began to sense that tranquillity could be part of my new, future identity. It certainly wasn't part of my past or indeed current one yet. She offered the idea of a softening, a slowing-down, based on her work in the water and as a woman in her forties too.

This moment of learning is especially precious to me now, because Nix, a mum of two young children, died unexpectedly the following July. Cancer gathered her up and swept her away, taking another person from my life during this messy middle bit. I still return to this moment on the beach and will do again as I get older; it was pivotal for me, and I could so easily have ignored it with my previous life mindset. It gave me a soft skill when mostly my personality, like many women's I knew, consisted of hard skills.

Midlife can be about seeking a new kind of peace in life. I'd found outdoor swimming, which had brought me adventure, cold water and a form of meditation I hadn't known I needed. But the swimming also tapped into the old me – the competitive, achieving, enduring bit of me. That Gen-X idea that if it wasn't hard to do, it wasn't worth doing. I think perhaps we all find this as we navigate the space between young and old.

As I aged I knew this addiction to the more manic side of life would be a hard one to beat. It wasn't like dry January, a matter of giving something up for a limited time. I was wired to achieve, to get stuff done, in almost every aspect of my life. Unwiring that would be a challenge. So many Gen-X women I talk to admit this too. This pattern of behaviour is mindless, rather than mindful.

But when someone with empathy, who has been through all this herself, points it out 15 minutes after meeting you, it does make you take a step back and re-evaluate what you're really looking for in a new you. How could it be so obvious to her, but not me?

I had to tap into something different internally. And Nix saw that, because she had seen it before in so many other women of my age. She was like a wise elder, one of those village matriarchs, or the Oracle in *The Matrix*. Through talking to Nix, mostly on WhatsApp, I began to sense this feeling of undoing – an unfurling.

The French-American artist Louise Bourgeois once held an exhibition that described the process many of us go through in this part of life as we find out who we could be. She called it:

I Do, I Undo, I Redo. Many of us are in the 'undo' bit, dismantling with discomfort who we were in preparation for the 'redo' bit, which feels a little way off initially but still exciting and optimistic.

Nix was nudging me through the undoing, asking me to examine the patterns, and also the language, that didn't work for me anymore. She was one of my external voices on the matter and it reminded me, as I often remind women when we chat about this, to stand back and look at what I was experiencing from the outside. Ask more questions and don't accept everything you see and hear as a rigid truth. Perhaps the absolute beliefs we hold can be changed, perhaps the limits we assume are real, or the limiting stories we tell ourselves are artificial, and we don't have to take any notice of them. When Nix died it was a stark and sudden reminder that you really don't know what is round the corner.

My swimming lesson with Nix was a life lesson. The water had brought many new women into my life, and now it had brought me Nix. Wasn't that the point? It wasn't about the actual sport, it was about the people, the places, being in the water. And how grateful I was that a pastime I had never considered – I mean, I couldn't do the front crawl until I was 47 – had brought me such gifts.

One of the last messages Nix sent me was her hoping that I was 'relaxing like an ever-unfolding flower'. 'Silly old hippy,' I thought before realising that this woman, whom I would sadly never see again, had had a profound and important impact on my life. If I could live it now like an ever-unfolding flower, wouldn't that be a wonderful thing? I dropped the cynical eye-rolls I'd normally have around this kind of behaviour and softened into that idea. What was the worst that could happen?

So the moral of this poignant story, aside from encouraging you to find your tranquillity in something that slows you down, is: find your women, because the one thing I know for sure, above all else in midlife, is that you need your female tribe. You won't get through this void, this pause, without them. It's like the bear hunt: you can't go over it, you can't go under it, you have to go through it. And you can't do it alone.

As therapist Julia Samuels told us on the podcast, the quality of our relationships predicts the quality of our lives; we are wired to connect. She said: 'Belonging is a vital foundation on which identity is built.'

I began to realise that people were becoming hugely more important than anything else as I aged, which sounds obvious, but in our speedy, mindless days we perhaps forget to nurture the people in our lives and focus too much on things instead – the house, the stuff, the job, the 'doing'.

An enormous urge to de-clutter comes to many midlife women too, like the one you get just before giving birth. You need a physical clear-out as much as you long for an emotional one, and, as all the stuff starts to go, the people take its place – the female friends.

So now is the time to find your tribe, even if that means shifting what you do, or connecting more thoroughly with the women already in your life in a more purposeful way. Let them see the parts of you that are changing. I think at this stage of life our identity is very much about who we know; we cannot underestimate the effect of those around us, and the vital need we have for them, and for social connection.

Here in midlife you are going to need to get vulnerable and ask for help, to be brave and seek out new women to support and guide you. I know, mad, isn't it? 'I've made a new friend' is something my 11-year-old would say after returning from a party covered in cheesy Wotsits.

Who would've thought you'd need to? But you really do; loneliness is only a heartbeat away, even if your life is filled with people and family on a daily basis. God knows mine is – just look at all those shoes and coats in our hallway. I am never alone, and yet these have been the loneliest of years for me.

I didn't expect to need new women now; I expected I'd be jettisoning those who were tricky and troublesome or fake and selfish, the time- and energy-sappers. I did not envisage bringing new women into the fold. But this new team of light really has been a life saver.

Which brings me to the longest-living trees in the world, the American redwoods. In my quest to sort my head out, to explore the living losses of midlife that I'd found out about and finally identified, I listened to a lot of podcasts (cliché that I am). And one day I found author Richard Powers being interviewed on *The Ezra Klein Show*. Powers is the Pulitzer Prize-winning writer of 13 novels; his voice is gentle and comforting, and he is a science and technology expert who challenges a lot of our current thinking. His book *The Overstory* is about a group of Americans brought together by the potential loss of giant redwoods due to deforestation – stay with me, I am getting to a lightbulb moment.

As I listened to Powers, he explained how it wasn't just the trees and the way they grew and lived as a community, with all the great history of our world running through their physical presence, that was extraordinary; it was also the community of fungi that lived on their roots and bark. This symbiotic relationship meant that the fungi helped keep the trees alive by delivering messages of need across the tree-verse. Apparently this happens with all trees within their species, but the redwoods are unusual because they talk to all trees and even offer help to those not of their own species. I don't fully understand the science of this, but I was drawn to the romantic notion that these trees have a network from another world looking out for them. And this is how I have come to view me and my new friends, the women from outside my world who have literally swum or walked into my life (walking is what we seem to do mostly after the Covid years). We are all interconnected like these giant prehistoric redwood trees, merging from outside our usual tribes, nurturing ourselves, nurturing others. Now, in midlife, we all seem to know our needs; women who are strangers often reach out with words of support too, all of us invisibly connected.

Perhaps we're all aware of our unique shared fate at this stage of life, so we have a spiritual affinity; we're rooted in each other's stories, there is an interbeing of us. It feels sturdy, it steadies me, and I really do need this common thread of experience in this moment. You will too, so look out for it, be open to new women, be curious and welcoming.

These women friends remind me that it is probably impossible to go back to my previous identity, to the way things were and still are sometimes in the back of my mind. They are there when moving through this undoing becomes uncomfortable, as it inevitably does because change is hard.

I met one of my new midlife friends in a small garden in Devon while I was on tour – as I like to call it – with my first book. I'd just been swimming in the sea (with another group of strangers I'd met virtually on Facebook – see? Women friends are everywhere!) and passed her chatting to another author on the front porch of a house they were sharing for one night for the literary festival. After that first meeting we went walking and talking and dipped in and out of the memories we had of London in the '90s. We had probably met before in those days. After our first walk she sent me an ironic text saying, 'Well, that was horrible.' I was noticing things and thinking, 'I must tell her about them.'

These new friends, the ones in the autumn of life, were like shafts of sunlight poking through stormy clouds on spring days, reminders of what I came to see as the unstoppable power of female friendship. And with friendships formed now in this era of easy connection (via the phone/social media) you can apply a lighter touch: a text, a picture. It doesn't have to go deep and be based on exhaustive confessional sharing. I don't need to know birthdays, or about children, mothers or lovers. I also feel like I want to present my most positive self to these new women in my life, which ripples across my day. Perhaps this is maturity? It makes me know how to handle friendship in a more empathetic fashion. And perhaps these new mates lighten the load of older, more complex friendships. They are shock-absorbers of my life, and I of theirs. Maybe this is Gen X's 'girl power' mantra coming of age?

It felt good to occasionally swim in a different pod. As we move through life we find friendship groups that suit the moment, and this midlife one felt so very welcome as I navigated this intense time. These women understood the assignment. I only knew them with the grey hairs and the laughter lines, and this was probably the version of them I needed, not the one that had come before. And they weren't interested in my work – that wasn't really relevant to our conversations, when it always had been with friends before.

They say you need 'radiators and listeners' in life; those are the women I treasured. The radiators I had had for years, and the new listeners who found me, together we could press our faces up against the glass of the future.

Make sure you are open and curious enough to find your new women, because they could be the people to pull you together when you feel like you are floating apart, when you have one foot on the dock and the other in the boat. Your stories will be different, but I can assure you the themes will be the same. And this is certainly the time of life when, as my teenage son, the gaming addict, would say, you have to 'choose your players' with care.

In my walks with my new Devon writer friend, we discussed the parts of ourselves we had hidden over the years as we were consumed with either our careers, marriage or motherhood. Those bits we squirrelled away because we didn't want to upset the apple cart, frighten the horses or impede our progress.

We may have hidden our reckless, carefree, possibly dangerous bits from our children as we parented them; we may have hidden our frivolous, fun-loving, impetuous or fearful side at work, or some of our femininity because we feared it would hold us back in certain jobs. We perhaps hid the parts we thought our partner might not like or might find unlovable in our relationships. I think I actually hid bits of myself in my childhood too, given the remote, traditional upbringing I received.

But these elements of us are still there, waiting in the wings to come out and be seen, to adapt and evolve. Or to be reckoned with. In psychology they seem to call this the 'essential self', and so it's worth exploring those parts again, in midlife, reviving them perhaps. After all, this is a time when you can choose who you want to be with greater freedom, show those bits of yourself to new friends and ask old friends to accept them. I think we can also be surprised by the bits we've kept out of sight. Perhaps we have become something we are not by accommodating others and compromising our personalities so much over the years? It's something I think women do far more than men, all this bending around people and muting of ourselves.

Maybe letting all these possible personalities back out is what makes it feel uncomfortable and messy now, like releasing a Pandora's box of Muppet characters. I certainly know it felt good to show some of my hidden parts to new people. I didn't feel the need to be funny all the time, as I had done in Act One of life. I didn't have to mention achievements or hide the chip on my shoulder about my lack of education! I could be prickly and let silence remain in conversations – something I'd feared before because I suspected it led to me being occasionally called 'tricky' at work, a term often used around women who don't respond in expected, acceptable ways. Tricky was OK with these new friends. They were strong enough to handle it, intrigued even. As the cloak of my career was left hanging on the door in new friendships, my main identity was not there to lean back on anymore. I could be myself.

One of the things my new female friends had in common was their ability to enjoy their own company comfortably. It could have been a coincidence, or perhaps I was looking for them, but this was the kind of woman I found. Being happy alone was something that had eluded me for most of my life; that hadn't been part of my identity up until now. When I talked about this with those friends I began to wonder if perhaps coming to London from Cornwall at such a young age on my own had meant I grabbed onto as many people as I could, like a lifebelt. I pulled them all around me all the time as a safety measure. It was always more fun, more secure, to be in a crowd, never alone with my thoughts. Early on in my career I was either in a giant open-plan newsroom or on the road as a reporter interviewing complete strangers. I found a long-term boyfriend immediately too.

One of my new friends pointed out that it wasn't 'normal' to leave home so young and go so far away, that a decision like that bore some investigation now further down the line. It would certainly have left a mark, been a difficulty that needed to be endured.

She also pointed out that my first relationship, with a man 13 years older than me, may not have been healthy; that, too, bore questioning. Perhaps there were legacy emotions to deal with?

I was gregarious and outgoing all the time after my initial year in London – maybe it masked fear and shyness? As the foundations of my identity fell away in my mid-forties, it seemed to me that maybe I was more of a loner than I thought; I had been as a younger child, constantly reading. Perhaps I was like a friend's tortoise, named Shelley (that's a *Blue Peter* reference, FYI. The mum kept buying Shelley a companion 'because she looked so sad' (we've all projected our feelings onto the family pet, haven't we?) and every time a new pet arrived to be around Shelley the tortoise somehow managed to disappear.

Perplexed by Shelley's disappearing acts, my friend and I googled this habitual behaviour and found out tortoises are solitary creatures; they don't want or need company. Shelley wasn't lonely, Shelley was just livid with all this enforced time spent in the company of others and wasn't prepared to compromise! She was a midlife woman! I don't think I am entirely a Shelley, a solitary animal; this is not the epiphany I had when I found that all my new friends seemed to share the talent of enjoying being alone. My awakening was that I had told myself a story about my identity based on all the squidging of it I had done as I aged. You can see how midlife fosters a confusing and contrary personality: I seemed to have learned that I could be happily alone by finding more friends.

My new women are a revelation to me. They are a reminder that in my forties and early fifties I still wasn't the person I would be yet – that we all have more growing to do, more people to meet. This was a hopeful thought during the midlife messiness, which often felt like the least hopeful of times. All this thinking about friendship would have looked illogical to me in my thirties and early forties. I would have questioned the idea of the redwoods' network because I wouldn't have foreseen this rough patch of life coming. It would have seemed a bit 'soft' to me. I would not have known the true value of female friendships and how much I was to learn from them.

I met Nadia, a yoga teacher, when I was writing a piece

for the *Sunday Times* about what a waste of time yoga was in 2019. So much contrariness in one sentence! Of all the teachers in London I could have interviewed, I found the one who at one point metaphorically pulled me out of the water during an emotional crisis with the strength and love of a human twice her physical size (she really is very tiny). I was drowning after a particularly traumatic family rupture and my new friend swiftly yanked me clear of the danger late one evening three years after we'd first met. 'I've never heard you cry before,' she said. 'I don't,' I replied, realising that wasn't normal either.

How joyous to have these new women here on the stands rooting for me. This is what my teen daughters might hashtag 'squad goals'. I had new allies, and I was open, honest and vulnerable with them. It was quite out of character.

These nourishing female friendships are the secret weapon of midlife, a silver lining, so I urge you to actively nurture the companions you have, to go out of your way to make these relationships good, and to find new ones to guide you forward. This is your barricade against the loneliness and confusion so many women tell me, and our podcast, that they feel. They will bring you cheer, make you less selfish and offer you comfort. They will also help you hone your ability to look at yourself from the outside in and question long-held truths.

Every now and again a thread will form on our podcast Facebook group about friendship, and I notice sometimes that a recurring theme is women feeling like their older friends are not there for them anymore, when they need them most. I occasionally step in to question this: are they not there or are you less available yourself? Have you ignored the offers of help because you feel uncomfortable showing vulnerability? Have you failed to ask for help, waiting for them to read your mind? Is your disappointment in them or is it in you? What's going on under this feeling of abandonment? Stepping back to question this can make you feel more open to asking more specifically for support; it can help you out of a rut.

These new friendships of mine have certainly made me more empathetic. I have noticed where I have been lacking in my old friends' lives, seen the support I failed to give, found the gap in the hedge through to a kinder way of being with those women I have known for decades (I hope . . . it is a work in progress). All this questioning of my own identity has made me more observant of the changing nature of the women around me who have been in my life a long time.

Science shows us that these connections are vital for your brain and your overall health. It also shows that these precious autumnal friendships will help you live longer. The bonds we form as we age are fundamental to our physical wellbeing. They hand us a safe zone where we can be ourselves or experiment with what our new selves could be. I have also reconnected with women I had only known in a work capacity before. I'd loved chatting with them on the phone during my career, and briefly in person, but had found a deeper connection with them now.

And, of course, my oldest friends have been a midlife lifeline, often in ways that are not always clear to me, but they have shored me up, consciously and subconsciously.

You need these women there, gently reinforcing your worth at a time when society deems it to be of less value. There is strength in numbers, confidence in voice after voice declaring the power of midlife women. And if you don't have this, you must actively seek it out, even though it will most likely be a harder task in midlife than it has been before. It's a form of gardening – planting the seeds of new friendships and watering the ones you have. Our groups on Facebook have brought the women of Gen X closer, and there is space on there to find your new women too, connect with others who have similar interests. But meet them in person too. This is not 'befriending', like a charity volunteer – it is opening up to new intimacies.

There is a saying that we are a parliament of all our selves, and this is never truer than in midlife, but I think we're also a parliament of all our friends, and those friends, old and new, are crucial to our future happiness. For me, it sometimes feels at this point like we're all standing on a pile of rubble after the earthquake of midlife. These wonderful women and I survey the wreckage of our pre-midlife identities, and when I ask, 'What do we do next?' they say, in the manner of the Rock surveying the rubble in *San Andreas*: 'We rebuild.'

8

The '90s Called – They Want Their Harem Pants Back

My wardrobe, probably more so than most, is a nostalgic line-up of pivotal points in my life: my past is literally staring back at me from the hangers, because clothes were such an integral part of my role editing fashion magazines. What I wore was always significant, even for a day spent in the office looking at page proofs, and I have been lucky enough to wear the most amazing clothes: pieces designed by the best of the best. I've been lightly stitched into a jacket by Domenico Dolce, I've had a couture dress made specifically for me, I've got Tom Ford bags (mostly leopard print; he knew I liked them), Stella McCartney PJs and Vivienne Westwood corsets. The Armani trouser suit I bought for a discounted price of £1,000 with my first *Cosmo* pay packet still hangs in the wardrobe 22 years later and I am still wearing the combat trousers I got when they were all the rage after All Saints wore them for their music videos. Mine are 19 years old. A silk grunge-era Alberta Ferretti '90s slip dress is quietly crumbling away on its hanger. There's a full-length Gucci maxi dress I was given as a birthday present that I am always worried I will trip on when I wear it and a formal black Chanel wool dress I just know the moths under my teenager's messy bed are dying to get at.

My outfits are my job identity. They are also a romp back in the fashion TARDIS, and when I go through the beautiful things I've collected over the years I am reminded of what a joyous adventure I have had and how lucky I have been to have landed in this career.

I was always careful not to get clothes confused with status in my day job, not to imbue the labels with meaning; just because I was wearing something designer didn't imply I was any better than a woman wearing something from the high street. I hope I avoided that kind of snobbery. And I was always aware that I'd come from a place where we saved up and bought our outfits from the Littlewoods catalogue or trips to C&A in Plymouth, so I never lost the joy of beautiful clothes. I borrowed much of what I wore during my career, so those pieces don't hang in my wardrobe today, but I bene-fited from hefty discounts as an editor and that stuff *is* hanging there, dripping in nostalgia.

But my life in clothes is a different story today. As I write I am wearing a pink dress I got in our local Oxfam. I don't need all the pieces I have gathered up over the years, and often I will feel overwhelmed by the volume of clothes, bags and shoes I have in the house. The weight of those memories is confusing as I try to work out what I like to wear now for stage two of my life, the bit where it might not matter so much anymore and where the realisation that you can't take any of these trinkets with you hangs heavily in the air on melancholy days.

Today I mostly buy pre-loved pieces because my teens are furious if I contribute to an industry that has a horrific ecolog-ical footprint; I'm too scared of them to bring a shopping bag containing anything new into the house! And rightly so. I'm proud of their commitment to saving the planet.

As I work out what to wear next (because I still love getting dressed), I have to come to terms with my changing shape. Midlife is not for the faint-hearted when it comes to looking in the mirror. And remember, we're Gen X, we have lived through a toxic culture of lookism. In the '90s newspapers were allowed to publish headlines about female TV presenters calling them fat; adverts were allowed to tell us men wouldn't look at us in jeans, they would only like us if we wore Pretty Polly fishnets. Any woman in the public eye was judged purely on her weight, shape and looks. Female victims of crime were described by their hair colour. Worse still, we were often told that what we wore was to blame for us being attacked. It was bad. So that's the context (which you probably know already) for many of our self-esteem issues as we head into our midlife years. You can't blame us for being concerned about how we will age physically.

But as an agent from your future (less *Men in Black*, more Woman Now in Brightly Coloured Patterns) I'm now going to give you notice of a few things that may happen to your face and figure in midlife.

Don't be alarmed, because, although this list is a bit worrisome, eventually it becomes evident that ageing is less about how you look and more about how you feel (and how you feel about how you look). I just think some advance warning of these changes is useful. And many of them will occur even for those of you who work harder than Gwyneth and any of the Jennifers (Aniston, Garner, Connolly, Lopez) to stay in shape. In my humble opinion, acceptance of these changes is crucial to your future stability and may require a new mindset around growing older.

But before we get to that, let's start with the list of what might happen so that you're not shocked, especially if you've already got a 'well none of this applies to me' mantra playing in the back of your mind.

Collagen hotline? Yes?
Well, where's mine all gone?

One morning, as you look in the mirror post-40, maybe post-45 if you're genetically lucky, you will notice that your skin has retained the creases of your pillow overnight. How annoying. Then, another day sometime later, you may look down and see that a suspicious loosening is occurring in the skin over your knees, and on your upper arms there's an unwelcome softening. Some of us notice small brown spots starting to appear on our face and hands, like little Marmite stains. Fine hairs make an appearance in places they didn't before. Your actual hair is thinner and takes longer to grow. Good God, some of us have now developed acne. The number 11 has etched itself almost overnight in between your eyebrows (which are paler, sparser, than ever before) and this makes you frown, making those lines worse.

All this 'looking' at yourself has also become troublesome because you find yourself continually squinting. Your eyesight is 'off'. How come you could read the instructions on your extortionately expensive hair-thickening shampoo yesterday but today it is tiny gobbledygook?

Why do brands do this, you wonder, market beauty help at midlife women and then make the type so small that only the under-forties can read it? Eventually you have to find your teenage daughter and ask her to read out the instructions for you, which comes with her inevitable chorus of, 'Mum, what the hell is wrong with you?' If you ask your son, he is kinder but says: 'Morag, man needs dem bins now, innit.'

Eventually you give in and acknowledge that your 'close-up' eyesight has gone so you have to buy some glasses. The first pair are nice prescription ones and you feel you look like Gloria Steinem in them, or Carrie from *Sex and the City*, but you lose them on day two at the shops and end up getting cheap supermarket ones so you can leave pairs all over the house. You also accidentally leave those in other people's cars, your best friend's handbag and anywhere you go on holiday – or in any room that has a telly in it because you can't read subtitles without glasses now, and you have to have the subtitles on because you can't concentrate on the telly if anyone is talking at the same time.

This midlife short-sightedness is alarming and causes as much havoc in the kitchen as it does in the bathroom when simple ingredients are unreadable. Tricky for a woman whose midlife gifted them a severe allergy. But you need the glasses in the kitchen because you must know how much hidden sugar is in everything due to the other surprising developments lower down your body. The tummy you sort of had under control until now isn't playing ball anymore. In fact, it is imitating a ball. Bloating or weight gain? Hard to say, but either way the appearance of tummy number two is extremely unsettling. And under your bra line on your back is a new layer of fat – extra padding in a place that did not tick the box for extra padding when the questionnaire was sent round.

All this is a slowly evolving and deepening mystery, especially the extra fat because you don't seem to weigh more . . . oh, hold on a minute, you do. How did that happen? You've barely changed what you eat in the past 20 years! 'What's wrong with me?' you may ask as all this occurs. It happens during the most confusing time, among all the other stuff that's going on in midlife, so you can't point the finger of blame at any one thing. You might have lost your mojo on all sorts of previously held good habits, because the fact is, you're holding up all the spinning plates and you haven't got time to do actual spinning anymore, like you did in your youth when that was a thing.

Whatever the changes are that you experience, it's all very disappointing, occasionally shocking and sometimes depressing, because your body holds echoes of your youth still; it holds the woman you were and may still think you are, and that's probably what we're all more worried about than the actual physical changes. This unexpected altering of the body feels a bit unfair; not fatal, just unfair. It's illogical, because we know it will happen, we just can't believe it when it does. Trust me on this, it is a wholly unbelievable situation despite the mountains of evidence to the contrary.

You get the drift: your body will change and, like empty-nest syndrome, like the sweaty insomnia, like the brain fog, like any of the other stuff you always thought other women were making a huge dramatic fuss over, it will almost certainly affect you emotionally more deeply than you anticipate. You could sit in the front row of every TED Talk on 'embracing the shape you are in' or 'changing the way you see yourself' and absorb all that body positivity, but I'm afraid you will still be alarmed by the grey hairs in your pubes and the way your hands suddenly look like they belong to a much older woman who lived a life in sunnier climes.

You can spout off about looking forward to 'hagdom', to being a creased and lined, wiser elder, but you'll still probably feel a melancholy twinge when a picture of you in your twenties is unearthed. You'll talk the talk about accepting your body now without the insecurities that may have warped the way you viewed your thighs in your twenties, but it's a bittersweet stage to reach because you will miss the elastin and collagen more than you think.

Often, in my late forties, I would stand in front of the mirror wondering who I was looking at. I'd see other midlife women pop up on my TV screen and wonder how long they'd been in make-up to change them so much. When Juliette Binoche appeared as her full, beautiful self alongside Colin Firth in some Netflix drama I couldn't believe my eyes. It wasn't the fact that she had aged – it had nothing to do with the wrinkles or the full head of grey hair – it was just that only yesterday she didn't look anything like that. In my mind, hours had passed, not decades, since she was La Binoche who had appeared in *Three Colours: Blue*.

Seeing all this happen around you, and to you, is alarming. It causes a quake in your own identity when the familiar looks of women you know – your cultural background noise – change as your looks change too. Your inner self is confused because she still feels the same. She looks like she did when she was 18 – or at least mine does. Or maybe 28. Younger, anyway.

I was quite disappointed with the sagging, mildly annoyed by the wrinkles, furious at the number-11 frown lines and inexplicably sad to see a new layer of body fat. I was keeping fit with swimming, yoga and all that other midlife malarkey – walking everywhere, weightlifting sometimes or going to Pilates like the good middle-aged woman I was. So it made me melancholy, this loss of the stretchier, smoother-skinned me, especially as the teenage clone of me was parading around in shorts and cut-off tops (my second daughter), confusing the computer in my head as to what year I was living through and berating me for plucking my eyebrows in 1984. I thought none of it would bother me, but I was wrong. It really did.

The point I am making is that these body changes are going to happen. They are going to mess with your mind and confuse your confidence. You'll lose around 30 per cent of your collagen during your perimenopausal years. Declines in oestrogen mean you'll lose elastin too. You'll even lose collagen from your gums, which changes where your teeth sit and therefore the shape of your face. You lose bone mass and muscle mass; your joints can start to ache as early as your mid-forties; you may even start making noises when you get out of a chair or put your feet on the floor first thing each morning. And while the jury is out on the direct links between hormone fluctuations and weight gain, the way we store fat does appear to change in midlife, so that thicker middle could become part and parcel of your new shape.

Obviously, everyone is different, so the list of potential changes is sort of endless. And, of course, some of us face illnesses that can change our bodies too, and then this worry about our wrinkles is really put into perspective. But these bodily changes are what they are, and coming to terms with them – your terms, in your way – is key.

I recall interviewing model, actor and fashion designer Sadie Frost about it, and she explained how she found herself completely mystified by the body changes. A former dancer, who was incredibly fit, who did Pilates and 35 years of yoga, who fasted and juiced, Sadie felt it was a huge challenge to come to terms with her new midlife body because it simply wasn't her. It wasn't who she was, she told us on the podcast. She was surprised to put on weight in her fifties. She had dealt with the extremes of postnatal depression in her life, suffered serious physical injuries and worked hard alongside bringing up four children at home, mostly alone. She considered herself 'tough as steel', she told us, having come from a childhood of poverty.

'I sailed through a lot of my forties. I'd had postnatal depression, been through divorce and the loss of my dad, and at these times I always felt I could cope. I am a strong person, I rarely cry. When you have gone to the extremes of mental health you have to manage the day to live it as best as you can.'

But then, she explained, something unexpected happened. 'Up to this point I had always looked good in all photos and then one day I [thought] OMG, what has happened to me? As soon as I turned 50 I put on weight, and suddenly I was at war with myself, and I had to learn to feel comfortable with it all and make some big changes. I had to change my diet, make sure I exercised well . . . It is a battle to feel confident and good and not have a horrible day thinking bad, negative things of myself.'

Like many women, Sadie felt as if she 'didn't do anything to deserve it; it just suddenly happens, and no one really told me'.

This war with weight is a subject we have tackled many times with experts on the podcast because the women in our midlife community ask about it relentlessly. I think perhaps we particularly obsess about weight gain because, at a time when we feel out of control, what we eat is one of the few things we *can* control – it is something we can alter.

Unfortunately, however, when it comes to the 'slow creep' (as Michelle Obama has referred to it) of the midlife middle, there is no magic bullet, no 'cure', no one thing to point the finger of blame at. The only general consensus from experts is that this is a time to avoid processed food, cut down on alcohol and sugar, and seek out a wide variety of fresh vegetables. Which you probably know already. 'Eat less, move more' is the mantra.

We've talked to women who have had great success in slimming to a size they are comfortable with on the more restrictive diets that reset eating patterns, but we've also talked to women who were made more unhappy by such rigid diets than they were by being overweight. Intermittent fasting has helped some (Professor Tim Spector's work with the ZOE project – a personalised nutrition programme – is helpful on how to do this). Many have found an exercise that keeps them trim, while others have simply eaten less and moved more.

It's such a personal choice, and there is not one thing that works for everyone.

We all know by now that excess fat isn't good for our long-term health, especially round the middle area. We know, too, that our nutritional needs and the way we store fat do change as we age, so taking time to address all this sensibly from a health standpoint is a good thing. For those on HRT who fear it has added to their weight gain, rest assured, a recent Swiss study showed that it actually lowers levels of dangerous belly fat – a fact Professor Tim Spector also confirmed on our podcast. But if you're worried, perhaps talk to your GP, and have a look at the books listed later (see page 236), which specifically deal with this conundrum. Experiment with what works for you, be patient with yourself and less disappointed, then focus on adding in some good habits, rather than taking things out and depriving yourself. Key to it all is adapting your mindset around your new size and shape.

You do you: it's mind, not body, that matters

I succumbed to the negativity of all the physical changes I was going through for a while because I had, like all of us, been indoctrinated into thinking that ageing is bad. It took a little while to gradually find a way out of that mindset and shut down that voice in my head that criticised what I looked like physically.

You can, of course, attempt to fight this by going high-maintenance on the body front with intensive exercise, or throwing money at all the modern fixes – or 'tweakments', as they're referred to – but you are still going to grow and look older, and the entrenched ageism in our society means you probably won't feel great about it. That is why the best line of defence is to shift your mindset around ageing.

This is far from easy. We've been told old is awful for women for so long it's hard to reprogram our minds to think more positively about it. We've done so many *Cosmo* quizzes, read so much *Bridget Jones*, bought so many diet books focused on quick fixes and generally lived a life of debit–credit eating and drinking that I sometimes wonder if this negative attitude is in our DNA, that it is unthinkable not to make a joke about the size of our thighs in shorts. You may feel fine about looking older, of course, but most of the women I meet 'hard agree' that body positivity is a young woman's game.

The language we use around ourselves, and the attitudes we hold, as we absorb the negativity around how society tells women to age, is important. With that in mind, a useful goal to help us reframe our attitude to ageing is to look 'better, not younger'. We're used to separating the mind and body, but they are one thing and it's time we started treating them holistically.

This is one of the reasons why I recommend outdoor swimming so highly – no one cares what they look like in that situation. You're so busy trying to stop your body going into hypothermic shock that the increasing droopiness of your midlife boobs as the tissue becomes less dense (yes, this happens) is the least of your worries. I find the attitudes of women around the lakes and on the beaches is good brain training. You get to see women of all shapes and sizes ageing actively. My swimming friends have, as someone put it on Instagram once, 'waved the white flag'; they have accepted their bodies as they are because if you stay on that path of not accepting it, of battling against it, you'll be on it forever, wasting precious second-life energy. Whereas if you choose to accept the body you are in as you age, you'll gradually find peace with it. Watching swimmers is proof that the body has one purpose, as the writer Donna Ashworth commented on Instagram: 'to see you safely through this adventure of life, to allow your spirit to reach full potential. That is it.'

I found that being among women who care less about the look and more about the spirit of a person after my lifetime in the fashion industry helped me reframe my attitude to body image. For one thing, I stopped talking about the changes after observing them. I didn't breathe air into my own negativity. Experts in adolescent mental health that I'd interviewed for my book on parenting teen girls told me that in an ideal world you'd never refer to looks or body image in front of your teenage daughter, never use the word 'beautiful' around them, to protect them from the complicated and never-ending tyranny of low body confidence. That's hard to do at home in reality, but it is easier to do around yourself, and it is an act of self-care. So after the initial shock of the changes, I just kept quiet about them. They weren't the most important thing about me, they were the least important thing, so there was no point wasting time on them. It took a while to come to a place where it wasn't a discussion point in my head, but at the same time I stayed fit, ate well, banked as much sleep as I could and was thankful I was on HRT.

Another thing that helped was discovering the work of Professor Ellen Langer, who is often referred to as the mother of positive psychology. Her in-depth research into ageing and mindfulness is important for us all to bear in mind in midlife. She is the author of *Counter Clockwise: Mindful Health and the Power of Possibility*, a book that asks: if we could turn back the clock psychologically, would it affect our physical health? She carried out several studies that seemed to show this idea to be true. One of the studies put men in their seventies and eighties into homes decorated from the era of their youth and asked them to live as if they had actually gone back in time. This appeared to turn the clock back for them physically; it helped with all aspects of their health, from hearing to weight loss. It didn't happen for a second group of the same age who were put in the same situation but told to just reminisce, rather than actually pretend they had gone back to their youth.

Langer's premise is that we need to stop operating on auto-pilot and open our minds to 'what is possible instead of clinging to accepted notions about what's not [possible], which can lead to better health at any age'. That sounds like good advice to me.

After all, age itself is a number, one we use to make all sorts of decisions and assumptions on what being a certain age means in the society we live in, but maybe none of those assumptions are true for us. Why should we fall for all the presumptions society lays at the door of a woman in her forties or fifties?

One can apply a bit of this thinking to body image and how we tend to value ourselves for our looks too. Can we make small changes in language and reorientate ourselves in our daily lives to feel younger and have a more positive mindset, Langer asks?

She famously studied a group of chambermaids and asked them to view their work as exercise rather than labour; they all lost weight and got fitter with no change in their daily activity. The mindset switch worked.

Obviously you're not going to get tickets to Manumission, pop on a boob tube and spray some Sun-In on your head before heading off back to 1989 to trick your body into looking younger, but a change of perspective will help you enjoy the ageing process more. Ignoring what we're told we should be in our forties and fifties is useful. I have tried it.

Langer's mantra is one of keeping a 'soft openness' to everything as we age, to accept that not knowing things (which often we can't) is a healthier, happier way to live. Making the most of every situation, whether it is a failure or a success, is crucial as we age, and Langer advises us to actively notice new things every day. See the sun come up sometimes, feel the fresh air – these small details of joy help us feel alive in our surroundings. They give us positive energy and make us more creative; they nurture our spirit. All of this, of course, is along the same meridian as the 'think well, act well, feel well, be well' idea.

I feel Generation-X women may have had an unhealthy focus on body image over the years. Imagine if you didn't ever have to say how old you were. Keeping that out of conversations would mean people didn't go ahead and make all sorts of assumptions about you based on what they believed a woman over 40 or 50 should say or do. So try to put your worries about what your body or face looks like on that list of things you refuse to think about in midlife, like the leaking tap in the loo, your kids leaving home for good, death . . . Put them there or tell yourself that unless you can say something nice about yourself, don't say anything at all.

Tweakments: a word

For me, the main problem was that it felt as if all these physical changes had happened without my consent, and that made me furious! I wrestled with this not because I wanted to look 25, or even 45, again, but because it was a shock and I didn't yet know how to style it out. But this change in body image can also be viewed as liberating. In my late forties I was sent by a newspaper to test Botox, to see if it could erase the wrinkly lines between my eyes that made me look more tired. It was fun to see the lines lessen (not disappear – it isn't a miracle wrinkle-eraser as it turns out), but I didn't have the urge to keep going back because I reasoned that something else would just start to bother me; the tide couldn't be held back. What I had to do instead was come to terms with this shift in my visual identity, acknowledge it and work out who I was with a changing face and body. It was my attitude I had to change, my disappointment I had to manage, not my lack of collagen. It was my optimism I had to fire up.

If you do want to try cosmetic procedures, though, and that makes you feel happier or more content, then good for you. If you want to know more, I suggest you follow expert Alice Hart-Davis, a journalist who has tried and tested many cosmetic procedures and has written *The Tweakments Guide* series of books on her findings. She first had Botox 17 years ago and believes it is a godsend for women wanting to feel better about the way they look. It is certainly becoming commonplace, with use among millennials increasing, many even starting under 30. We interviewed Alice on the podcast and she seemed very matter-of-fact about her treatments, undergone to 'stave off the ravages of time', as she put it. I think this area of maintenance comes under the 'each to their own' category. I don't judge any women for their choices. As with anything, just make sure you are doing it safely.

Find your style: some thoughts

Maybe this is where I should offer some practical advice on style as we age. Mindset change aside, I have spent a lifetime in the fashion and beauty world, so I should have learned a few things to help you develop your new 'better, not younger' mindset.

Firstly, there are no rules. Dressing for your age is a ridiculous concept. Nothing is ever one size fits all and we live in a time when looking your age as a woman seems a radical thing to do. It's about experimenting and being curious, trying new things and deciding not to feel selfish or shallow for investing time and cash in your outfits.

Around the age of 48 I started to look for visual templates of women who seemed to have aged with elegance and confidence and whose style I liked. For me, those women included

Sharon Stone, Viv Albertine, the retailer Linda Fargo, model Inès de la Fressange, Jennifer Saunders, Michelle Obama, Annie Lennox, Emma Thompson, Viola Davis and Jamie Lee Curtis, among others. These were women whose style I liked, but you may have a completely different set that you admire. Find pictures of them and see what it is you like about the way they look or dress. What can you adopt from the way they have aged, or how they dress their midlife bodies?

When it came to my own style, I wanted something uplifting on the clothes front. I needed to step out of the career 'uniform' that had held me in place for decades and find a new one. So I stopped wearing so much black and opened the door to bright, block colours and prints, which I had run screaming from for years. I got rid of underwired bras – threw them all away – and discovered the bralette, an altogether easier thing to put on after a swim.

As I softened in midlife, so did my wardrobe; it morphed into something I think you could perhaps call modern comfort. I'd often wondered why more mature women wore so much colour and big jewellery, and as I aged I realised it was because they felt liberated from sartorial expectations. They went for choices that made them feel more positive, gave them more energy. It was an act of self-care for them to dress this way, and it works. I highly recommend a colour injection at this stage of your fashion life, and adopting a positive mindset: caring about what you wear is not self-indulgent or frivolous. It is the very basis of your identity; it is something to embrace and enjoy.

However, I notice from our community that a river of fear still appears to run through ordinary women of my generation when it comes to clothes (and colour) – I hear about it all the time. 'This won't suit me', 'I can't wear red', 'I need a huge belt to cover my waist' – we have a head full of rules that are meaningless and factually incorrect, which should be challenged every day. The only one worth sticking to is, 'Does it have pockets?' because pockets are good. Here are one or two more thoughts that may help you:

~ Invest in some good-quality underwear that matches and fits properly, then start to wear what makes you feel comfortable over it.
~ Use getting dressed as a way to make yourself feel positive about the day ahead, instead of reverting to previous notions of looking good at work, dressing for your job or attracting the interest of men. Enjoy 'creating a look' for yourself each day, and refuse to become intimidated by clothes. Go for items that make you smile when you put them on. A giant trying-on session of all the things you'd previously shunned may be worth investing time in too. Take it seriously and plan a day for it.
~ Accept that you'll have to let go of stuff – I had a good run with heels, but they are not for me anymore, even though I am only five foot two.
~ Allow yourself to be persuaded out of your adherence to old rules. For example, I love a jumpsuit, but my podcast co-host Trish refused to wear them until I made her try one. Now she is a convert! Sure, adjustments might be necessary – the jumpsuits of my past were all structured; now I go for less hard-edged versions (rather like myself) – but that's all part of the fun.
~ Dress your shape, don't hide it. Accentuate the waist, whatever size it is – wear high-waisted; go for belts.
~ Experiment with things and try to buy the best mid-price quality you can.
~ Never buy cheap jewellery.
~ Tweak things to fit. I get a lot of pre-loved fashion taken

in or up at my local dry cleaner's, which is affordable if you buy second-hand in the first place.

~ Never shop for a single piece; shop for whole looks, and by that I mean buy things that go with other things in your wardrobe. So don't get anything new unless you know what you will wear with it.

~ When it comes to jeans, finding the right pair seems to really bother midlife women. It is all about the height of the waist and where the pockets are (skinny jeans don't suit anyone, IMO). A higher waistline is more flattering on most women. The top button should sit on your natural waistline, and I go for darker washes as I think they are more stylish.

These are just some ideas to help you navigate style in midlife, but really, you can make your own rules now. I am certainly a little 'dressier' as I age – I put in more effort, not less; it makes me feel good and I like to think people notice. I don't keep anything for 'best'; I wear items all the time even if I never leave the house. I am not suggesting older women should go for attention-grabbing outfits, more that they can avoid boring choices.

I also 'had my colours done' – a very '80s concept – for the podcast and discovered that lime green, brighter pinks, red and brighter oranges really suit me. Black does not, which confirmed my suspicion that I'd been hiding behind it at times.

As I started to wear these new colours, which had never had a place in my wardrobe before, my persona evolved. I still wore trouser suits when I was out and about, but this time in bright colours. And as I cleared the wardrobe of clothes that realistically I would never wear again (sold on eBay or given to charity shops) I felt a sense of freedom. I think if you haven't worn it for six months to a year, it has to go to a better home where it will be more appreciated (like hamsters).

Losing all this 'stuff' felt like clearing a blockage for me. I felt a weight lifted off my shoulders, as if I was able to formally say goodbye to the fashion part of my career. I felt relieved of the pressure of looking right, which had in some ways followed me around for much of my career; now I could wear what I wanted. It will, of course, be a different story for you, but the lesson is to be mindful of making positive changes in your wardrobe. We're all grown-ups and we know it's not about 'the dress' but about the 'woman in the dress'; however, when people notice you at a time when you may feel invisible, as if you are fading away, it does give you a lift. A new you may well need a new look, and it's not shallow to indulge in the joy of clothes.

Of course, I acknowledge that it is easier for me to work out what to wear than for most – I have been lucky enough to work with some of the world's best stylists and I have always loved clothes. They may not be your thing at all – you might be perfectly happy in a onesie teamed with UGGs, and that's OK, but don't underestimate how wonderful it is when you feel happy as you get dressed in the morning. It's another way you can bring a playful new attitude into your midlife.

Beauty: some thoughts

There are some basic beauty ideas for midlife too, I think, if you fancy knowing them:

~ Spend your money on your hair and your nails. Looking groomed is always down to this, really. And know that going grey – full grey – is no longer seen as giving in – just look at Andie MacDowell. If it makes you feel good, do it.

~ Change your skincare routine to adapt to your skin as it changes with age. What worked in your twenties won't work now. You may need to investigate products with vitamin C in them or retinoids for night-time, and you'll need a better body moisturiser, as most women's skin gets much drier in midlife. Sleep is your biggest skin boost, as well as more water, less booze (boring, but true). I've popped a list of places and experts who can help in the back of the book because it is worth spending time on getting that right.

~ If you do yoga or Pilates your posture will be better and your breathing, which all helps your skin, and helps you sleep, which helps your skin.

~ Get a good dentist and look after your teeth.

Ultimately the goal is to get to a place where you feel happy and healthy as all these changes happen. So for God's sake wear that bikini, feel the warmth of the sun on your body and enjoy the water on your skin. As a woman who had been given only a few months to live in her fifties told me, life is too short not to.

101 Things Only Midlife Women Know: You're a Gen Xer If . . .

~ I say 'Shazza' and you immediately think blue soup.
~ You still believe Wagon Wheels are for posh people.
~ I say *Bagpuss* and it makes you smile.
~ You say 'I'm going to record that' out loud about telly programmes.
~ You know the *Swap Shop* number (01818118055)
~ You fancied David Soul in the cardigan photo-signing phase. This sentence makes no sense to millennials.
~ Findus Crispy Pancake is one of your passwords.
~ You get the Heardle in one second when it is a Wham! song.
~ Your husband says 'Joooooooon' very loudly the day May comes to an end.
~ On every humid summer evening you mumble, 'It's like *Tenko* in here.'
~ Your early cultural references start at Margo Leadbetter and end at Gordon the Gopher.

9

'Every Now and Then We Fall Apart': The Secret Shame of Midlife Women and What You Can Do About It

I'm waiting in the breakfast room of Paris's Le Meurice hotel on a sharp, sunny day. It's fashion week. Le Meurice is the hotel where Salvador Dalí waltzed up and down the giant foyer with his pet ocelot when he lived in the presidential suite. The bar is chic, as it was then; the breakfast room not so much. It's a bit boring until my guest, the French designer Isabel Marant, walks in. All smiles and no make-up, she strides across the room carrying a glistening white motorcycle helmet and wearing a soft black leather jacket. Her long grey and brown hair is artfully styled-not-styled. Her eyes are twinkly.

Marant is cool, we all know that. It's her brand – loose boho pieces or grey jeans and rough-edged tees; big logo sweatshirts that somehow don't look cheap or like sportswear.

She's the designer of the perfect suede ankle boot. Every vintage hoarder in the fashion world has Marant on their permanent eBay watch list. I'm a few years younger than

Marant, but I feel older and old-fashioned in comparison, too formally dressed and slightly embarrassed by my uptight Britishness. She is coming to meet me so we can discuss a piece for *ELLE*. She's the exotic ocelot and I am the boring British tabby cat.

I order eggs (she just has a black coffee) and we talk about her cabin in the mountains – it's got no electricity or hot water. She loves it there, and she isn't being pretentious, just matter-of-fact. 'Exactly the kind of older woman I want to be,' I think as I watch her. I don't see many Marant-like role models around me, but it feels like she's at the right place on the dial as I am tuning into my midlife fantasy of what comes next. When she leaves we walk out together onto the busy Rue de Rivoli. I expect her to hop onto a scooter with her helmet; instead, she mounts a massive motorbike. It's so heavy the tarmac almost dents as she hauls it off its stand. And when she starts the engine the noise is like something out of a Hells Angel movie. As she rides off I notice she is wearing five-inch white stiletto shoes.

'I've just seen the woman I want to be when I get older,' I tell my Gen-X WhatsApp group. 'This is what I want my fifties to look like,' I think.

Isabel seems neither young, nor old, but the reality for me is so different. I cannot even work out how to feel like Marant looks and acts as I get older; that easy, stylish confidence is elusive. There's a huge disconnect between what I thought midlife would be and what it actually is. And that delusion is part of the problem. Our problem, maybe.

Where's the confidence born out of a lifetime of experiences, good and bad, that everyone talks about? Where's the patience, the ease in dealing with everyday situations that I expected? It's more than an anti-climax, it is a bloody let-down!

That's what this middle bit is: a totally unexpected outcome.

The phrase 'I bet you didn't think that would happen?' becomes the refrain for those of us who get lost here. I hear it over and over as I stalk the Facebook groups, scroll through the Gen-X WhatsApp conversations, listen to the stories of women over 45, or younger in some cases. I hear it from those who don't come from where I come from, those going through entirely different experiences at this stage of life. We really didn't think this wobble in our identity would happen.

'Why would you?' as Ruby Wax asked on our podcast from the vantage point of her sixties. 'I mean, if you really believed you were going to just die someday, you'd never get out of bed in the morning. It's the same as childbirth too. We could tell you how midlife was going to be, but you wouldn't believe us anyway.'

So here I am. I could never get a big motorbike off its stand without getting trapped under it and I can't wear heels anymore because I have arthritis in my feet. My wistful Marant daydream is just that: a soft fantasy, because the reality is confusing and unclear.

What women tell me

I am not alone in all this confusion. As well as talking to friends and to women on the podcast, I also set out to interview women who occupy a very different place to me as I started to write this book. I wanted to get a complete picture of what they were going through too. I wanted to hear from women who were none of the things I am, and so I sought them out. I loved talking to them because they made me feel like I belonged to something. I wasn't going slowly mad on my own, and it *was* OK to do a bit of navel gazing around all these new feelings.

Because we're not moaning, you understand. None of us is moaning, not even the wonderful woman who signed off her email with 'it'll be a cheerful chat, I'm not miserable all the time', after telling me her much-loved husband of 17 years had dropped dead of a heart attack out of the blue one day. (Side note: Your world collapsed, you and your young children were devastated by grief just six weeks before Covid struck, it's unimaginably sad. You CAN moan.)

In this chapter I tell their stories anonymously in more detail. All their experiences are, of course, phenomenally different, but this thread of loss – the loss of identity and confidence mainly – and confusion is common to them all. These losses are what therapists refer to as 'living losses' and they are their own kind of grief.

As one single mum told me: 'Before now, each decade ahead was easy to see – they mostly looked appealing, fun even, an adventure – but at 45 I couldn't see what was ahead anymore. I couldn't even peek round the corner. I was just staring at a blank wall.'

The realisations of the women I spoke to were fascinatingly diverse, but there was a commonality in them wanting to 'get it done' or push through and sort things out, no matter what or how adversely, harshly or horribly it affected them, from cancer diagnoses to many forms of grief. Many could only admit to an unravelling in retrospect.

Few seemed to find compassion for themselves in their situations. And the moments when they did discover this unexpected internal empathy for their own experiences were quite a revelation to them, and for many a helpful turning point.

I was amazed by how 'tough' these women from all different backgrounds and ethnicities expected themselves to be, how hard they were on themselves as a tsunami of change swept into their lives. Many were perfectionists, setting themselves unrealistically high standards in every area of life. 'Jesus, ladies, give yourself a break!' I wanted to yell as we chatted, especially to the woman whose monstrous perimenopausal period started out of the blue in the middle of a job interview at 49.

'So unprofessional,' she tells me while I struggle not to blurt out, 'It's not your fault!' She was going for a job she didn't even know if she wanted. She was older than the other candidates, patronised by the panel who interviewed her and then, to top it off, her body threw her a curve ball that washed away the last remnants of her career confidence.

'In the two previous interviews I had overprepared,' she tells me. 'And I was then so nervous I couldn't articulate how experienced I was for the roles. In one I looked up at one point and the man on the panel had fallen asleep. I was terrified that I had reached an age in life where people fell asleep when I talked to them.'

During her next interview, for another job she was overqualified for, she had a hot flush. 'I was sweating profusely and suddenly I was also having my period. I shuffled backwards out of the door in my dark trouser suit, mortified. I was in the middle of a presentation.'

As we chat this through, I notice we're both laughing hysterically – it's like a scene from a sitcom entitled *101 Horrific Things That Happen in Midlife That No One Told You About*.

JC, as I will call her, is a civil servant and says she had to 'chalk the interview up to experience'. Her story chimes with so many others I have heard from women trying to forge a career path in midlife but feeling a secret shame around it.

'I had felt so side-lined at work, as if I was on the scrap heap. I looked around me and couldn't see any middle-aged women. I knew I was off the boil, but I needed to get a job for my mental as well as financial wellbeing. I still wanted to be part of the fabric of life.'

For JC the process was 'horrendous', 'demeaning', and the effect was cumulative: 'My confidence fell off a cliff, I'd lost out on promotions, I couldn't find a new role. I couldn't work out who I was . . . I was harking back to my thirties when I was so ambitious. I could take on anything then and now I had lost the ability to articulate any of that. I felt so insignificant . . . At the same time my dad, who was my biggest support on the career front, was dying, and suddenly he was gone.'

As a mum of three, JC is well aware that if she'd worked in the private sector she might never have found a role. Now she heads a small civil-service research team.

'I still sit at work and watch teams of younger men getting promoted ahead of me and the older women I work with, but I know I am lucky to be here.' She sighs. 'But for ages I just wasn't myself. I was so angry and there were moments when I thought I was about to become a basket case and I would end up divorcing my husband and leaving my family.'

She sorted out her perimenopausal symptoms by going on HRT and says she has changed her attitude to accommodate a new midlife mindset.

'My mum is 86, she is a formidable woman and I see her and it makes me really want to make the most of all my time now. I have this attitude each day where I get up and say this is a new day, let's change what we don't like, stop doing what we're not happy about, let's tap into the energy of a new start and make it good.'

This notion of time running out is often the driver for positive change among the women I have talked to – it is the phantom breathing down all our necks during our big pause in midlife. This is the time when some of us are just sort of 'noggling' through. 'Noggle' is an old dialect word that means just about get through something but with great difficulty, and that's what 48 to 51 felt like to me – so much noggling, as time sped up. But I have to tell you that after 50, I was not in the mood for any more noggling.

Many women I talked to also had a feeling of shame around how successful or capable they used to be, and how that didn't fit with who they were now; it was a secret they kept from everyone. They suddenly felt irrelevant and in one woman's words 'so useless' that they didn't dare mention their amazing earlier successes out loud. 'People would be incredulous if I talked about how well I did in my job; they would think I was making it up,' one told me. This shame around our past is unhelpful. We're made up of all the women we once were, so keeping those successes alive is imperative if we are to maintain our feelings of self-worth.

It's something that comes more into focus with the onset of the brain fog many of us experience in perimenopause – forgetting words, names, how to do simple tasks. My memory loss made me feel ashamed and as if I was at the beginning of a long, slow decline into incompetence after years of what I felt was razor-sharp focus.

Obviously many midlife women I spoke to had retained their quick thinking, but a lot had lost it in the hormone storm. Brain fog is not permanent (HRT reversed mine) and we're still as good at our jobs as we used to be, we just have to find the way to work around the memory lapses. Often reducing stress and getting healthier helps, as being overwhelmed affects our ability to retain information too.

But menopause and perimenopause have remained unmentioned for so long that it's a difficult conversation to start, and we have accidentally colluded in the denial of its existence at work. The midlife wobble we have derails us but it doesn't need to. We can avoid the shame if we address it early enough. And it is important we do that.

After all, women over 50 are the fastest-growing work demographic in the UK, so employers would be wise to offer them the support they need. When gender equality charity the

Fawcett Society conducted a landmark study of menopause and the workplace in 2022 for Davina McCall's award-winning Channel 4 documentary *Sex, Mind and the Menopause*, it found that the majority of women (77 per cent) had at least one menopause symptom that was 'very difficult', while 44 per cent experienced three or more symptoms they called severe. The same percentage of menopausal women in employment said their ability to work had been affected.

Despite this, 8 in 10 menopausal women said their workplace had no basic support in place for them – no support networks (79 per cent), no absence policies (81 per cent) and no information-sharing with staff (79 per cent). Nearly a fifth – 21 per cent – of women who have to wear a uniform or abide by a dress code for work say it is uncomfortable given their symptoms, rising to 28 per cent among working-class women, while 81 per cent of menopausal women agreed that every employer should have an action plan on the menopause.[10]

The stats speak volumes for the women who have largely been silent. Fear of speaking out and this odd shame around losing our skills have been actively hindering the women of Gen X in the workplace, obliterating their confidence.

Being heard

One day I listen to Deborah Levy on Radio 4's *Woman's Hour*. She is in her sixties. She says that it is important to write about the things we don't understand in life. When you start to explore the bit between not understanding it and understanding it, then it delivers the coherence you might be searching for, which is what it felt like interviewing all these lovely midlife women. This is how we get to understand what is happening to our identity as we age, by exploring it and talking about it. I don't think voicing our needs out loud is dangerous for working women, as some commentators say (they think it portrays us as weaker); it is about defining a hopeful and positive path back to ourselves, or to a new version of ourselves, and offering advice for younger women at work.

We are perhaps the first generation to publicly discuss all this. We're on TV, radio and podcasts talking it through, and we're beginning to understand the bit we didn't know about before. The path through stage two is being better defined, and we're the cartographers. We're getting the help we need and learning that it is possible to retain and improve all our skills, to package them up alongside a lifetime of experience, and offer wiser versions of our youthful selves. It is only through other women's stories that we can understand this feeling of shame and being an imposter or fraud, and therefore stop it setting off the spin-cycle of dispirited disappointment in so many women. Discussing it helps solve our problems; it puts us back on track.

Sam, a mum of two, now in her early fifties, is a prime example of a high-achieving woman who has lost all her confidence in midlife. For Sam, a former long-haul airline pilot, the loss of her identity now she is retired, along with her extreme coping capabilities (I mean, can you imagine being able to fly an actual plane?), has been a life quake.

'I am terribly lost,' she tells me. 'My marriage is all but over, it's irreparable; I lost my dad when I was in my early forties, [and] I feel as if it has all been downhill since then . . . I never mention I could land a 747 out loud because today I can barely park the car. I don't see that me in the me [now] at all. I see it in one of my teenage daughters but never in me. I don't think I fit in anywhere. I feel as if I am a different person entirely and I find that scary.'

Sam is on HRT after listening to our podcast and watching Davina McCall's documentary and says she believes 'a rebirth' of sorts is possible for her over time, but right now she is stuck. I think she knows her inner strength will start to grow as she gets her voice back, but I can see how much of a shock this has been for her. She's 'battling to be me again', she says. She's had therapy, got fitter, found her tribe of mums. She's bought a vibrator. All this has planted the seeds of hope in Sam's life. She knows divorce may be imminent, that time is precious and that she needs to move forward. I want to swoop in and show her a movie of her past to fuel the energy she'll no doubt need to move forward because, like many, she faces so many choices at her midlife crossroads that she never thought she would. She doesn't feel the way she envisaged, which is a refrain I consistently hear.

Jo also tells me she feels rudderless. In her early fifties, she has now passed the age her mum was when she died and is in free-fall at the unexpected emotions of midlife. Primary among them is a crisis of confidence in her career.

'I don't have the willingness to be that tigress at work anymore,' she explains. 'I was ruthless as a young woman at work, but not now . . . I've been made redundant now . . . my boss wouldn't let me go at first, but my mindset was wrong, I wanted to leave. I had this idea of going off to live alone in the countryside, to maybe study again, just to get out of this high-pressure job. I wanted an escape.'

Jo's job had always been a source of strength and pride for her, and now it was becoming the opposite: 'I always felt invincible at work until one day I didn't, I wanted to disappear. I am now in a place where I genuinely don't know what to do next. I am half-heartedly applying for jobs, and I work in tech, so this is a nightmare process. Everyone is younger by many years and for one job I had not one, but two interviews where I had to video myself and ask myself the questions. It's a living hell . . . I'm punishing myself to test if I still have that edge.'

Jo is childless by choice. She is also now single after a complicated relationship ended. What she is looking for, she says, is
a sign from the universe – 'the thing that will take me forward'.
The question is, where?

'In a way I have been ticking boxes all my life. Now I am
not in one. The "what next?" question is defeating me. I made
this choice, though. I stepped out of the job willingly.'

I can sense that Jo feels she has failed somehow. She mentions
also that her dad died recently, and she had been nursing him
through his illness. She is finally on HRT, which has helped with
her physical symptoms, but emotionally she is still in turmoil.

'Before my mum died in my twenties I had the attitude that
I was going to make the most of every minute, live life at
100mph, and I went off and travelled the world in my twenties.
I don't want to do that now, so I can't work out how to feel.
I am in this blank space and learning to sit with all these feelings. I know better times are ahead – I have been listening to
all the podcasts, read the books that tell me so – now I just
have to figure out how to move forward, not sideways.'

A whole new career

For many of the women I chatted to, the shock of midlife was
that they didn't end up taking the path they had planned to
after the big job, the mothering or the marriage. Sometimes
these long-held dreams lose their appeal when the time comes
to make them a reality. Clare, also in her early fifties, has three
kids, and the last is about to leave home.

'I began to question my goals in my late forties. I have had a
good life, lovely family, great career running businesses I had set
up. My husband and I planned to cash it all in and head off
travelling. To see the world, free of the responsibility of work
and family.

'But when he said, "OK we can go now," this year, I didn't want to. It was a surprise to feel like this . . . I felt I had been focused on everyone else's needs for so long and was suddenly more curious about my own. And wandering the world looking at temples didn't appeal, even though that had been the plan all along. I just had another itch to scratch.'

The nature of that itch, however, was difficult to define at first. 'I had a fear of retirement, a fear of slowing down. I think it is a fear of lack of purpose. I am not bothered about ageing – I am on HRT, I dealt with all the physical issues and emotional ones that came with that, and I am not overly focused on [the] empty nest.

'It was a surprise for me to feel this way about travel. My husband had packed our bags, they were in the hall, but in that moment I said no. I wanted to be around for the kids popping back at weekends, I wanted to carry on working, and I also had this feeling I wanted to "give back" . . . I think maybe I wanted to feel needed too.'

Clare has now begun to train as a therapist and plans to work pro bono for those who need it in her community. She's also started to foster abandoned puppies, and the effect has been transformative.

'I was kind of chaotic and ditsy in my younger days and now I feel as if I am totally focused. This is the new me. I am a different kind of person in midlife. As soon as I made the decision, I suddenly felt happy about life, enthusiastic. I didn't want to go away and miss all the good things in my life I had here, if that makes sense. I didn't want to start again, I wanted to help out here. I sort of diverged from what was expected of me by the rest of the family.

'For so long my job was about earning money for us all and now I have done that I feel like success has to be measured in another way. I was "work hard, play hard" then too. Now I am not. I have to space out any socialising with any work needs. Slowing it all down has made life feel easier for me. I have maybe 30 years ahead of me of feeling useful and working, so I feel like I want to get as much done as possible.'

It's refreshing to chat to Claire. She's got a quiet 'I am not for turning' tone about her and I can imagine her husband was quite baffled when she refused those plane tickets and filled the house with small fur balls. She's crossed that void into stage two of her life, and is not stuck in the honey-like stillness many of us encounter – a place you really should only sit for a short while before taking positive action to move on.

A deeper love

Maria is deep into her second act after stepping out of a troubled 25-year marriage to start all over again. A high-flying banker, with twin 19-year-olds (one of whom has had a serious illness for most of her young life), Maria now has what looks like a fairy-tale ending, but her story hasn't been without great sadness.

'I was sleepwalking through my life for the longest time,' she tells me. 'I did it for the right reasons – for the children, I was trying to be a good mother – but the partnership had been over physically and emotionally for a while.'

As the family's main breadwinner, Maria stayed married to keep life consistent for the family, but she was sacrificing her own fulfilment along the way.

'My husband wasn't active in our relationship; he didn't contribute financially and he wasn't helpful or supportive. It wasn't a harmonious place to be. When I left I knew I was leaving something that I didn't want – it was a very lonely place. I am and always have been an optimistic person, but I could see our problems were not going to go away. Things would not have changed if I had not changed them.'

145

Maria opted for divorce, at first trying to keep everyone living in the family home, but she recognised that that was untenable and eventually decided to start over.

'I had to step out of the routine to acknowledge the reality of what was going on at home,' she explained. 'I had developed a very low self-esteem in my marriage. I couldn't help but think I deserved the way I was being treated, but I also knew I couldn't hide all these feelings from the kids, so it was time to go.'

She says the decision to part with her husband was 'terrifying', but, interestingly, she also tells me that the thing she thought would be her greatest challenge actually turned out to be her greatest strength.

'Once I had worked out that "staying for the kids" was a nonsense, I also realised that being in total control of the money was liberating. I kept thinking how awful it would be to be alone at this stage of life, then I realised I was already alone.'

While making this seismic life change, Maria also experienced upsetting perimenopause symptoms, which she sorted out after the divorce. The split meant she could finally address all the routines she had clung to.

'From the age of 30 to 40 I was just getting through, but I feel that now, five years after the divorce, I am living again. I was so lost, constantly wondering, "Who am I?" And then after the parting, I had to find a new identity and I got to decide what that could be.'

And how. Right now, Maria is packing her bags for her new job in Lisbon with her lover of the past three years, whom she has just moved in with.

'I met him on a dating app,' she tells me. 'I wasn't looking for "the one" or for a partner at all, just [testing] out what a date may be like after 25 years of not having been on one . . . This bit of life feels like a complete rebirth for me. Not at work

– there I know I am just hanging in until I am not as relevant as the younger person underneath me – but at home I am on the cusp of something new.

'It's crazy, and five years ago if you had told me this would happen I just wouldn't have believed you. I am energised by life now. I feel so healthy, and it feels as if I have created a second chance for myself. And I could so easily have stayed, and not done that.'

This has been such a dramatic shift for Maria, an unlocking after an unravelling. 'I took a huge risk, and it has paid off for me, for which I am really thankful and grateful, and I also know I am lucky to have my health. I was so afraid of what would be round the corner, but I knew I couldn't live under that fear. I knew I had to eventually be true to myself, and that is when things started to change.'

Her renewed sex life has perhaps been the icing on the cake for Maria, a shy woman who has overcome her reticence about this aspect of life simply so other women can have some sense of what is possible.

'We have to share this stuff,' she tells me. 'Sex has been amazing for me. I was in a sexless place for years and years, and then I found a partner who saw me as feminine. I didn't feel it at first, but he saw me as a whole woman and we'd have these crazy dates with lots of sex. We'd meet in hotels until I was sure I could bring him home to meet my children and it felt so fun, so spontaneous. He liked my body as it was – the shape I was in was fine for him. I am not a small yoga-bunny type of woman, but that didn't matter, and that was utterly liberating for me and gave me a confidence I had not had before.'

Maria's story is truly remarkable. It's good to hear that such an uplifting outcome is always possible in this confusing part of life.

Maureen got married in her late thirties and embarked on a career adventure – she headed to LA with her husband for a job in personnel for a huge corporation. Her work days were 12 to 14 hours long and the stress was immense, even though she loved the job. At the same time, she suffered several miscarriages, and then she decided she'd had enough. Aged 46, she quit the job she loved and decided to retrain as a nutritionist.

'On reflection, I wasn't being logical. I wasn't myself. It was a crisis of identity,' Maureen, now in her early fifties, tells me. 'I just wanted a way out of the stress, to get away from such an intense environment. It was quite OTT to quit completely and do something totally different.' We laugh for a good 10 minutes about why she didn't just ask for some time off, but we both acknowledge that this perimenopause phase of life often tosses logic out of the window, drama queen that she is.

'Looking back, I can see that I just wanted to be a softer person. The job wasn't the issue in many ways; I was the issue . . . I put on a coat of armour to go to work every day; it was all about achievement for me. About winning. I was a type-A person. The status I got from my job and from the title attached to it seemed to be the most defining thing, and to combat that I think I just abandoned it all together, which was a huge shock once I had done it.'

This was a drastic step for Maureen; she was leaving the safety of her job and the status it gave her to willingly jump into the void, and it was a scary place to be.

'I had taken a leap of faith, but it was extremely unsettling for me at the beginning. I show up at work now as who I am, no armour, but in my previous life I was addicted to that manic way of being and it has been hard to shake off . . . Even when I do sports I throw myself at them with a high sense of perform- ance, and I had a trainer say to me recently that I would achieve more if I slowed down, if I was more compassionate about myself and to my body. It is such a learning curve.'

Like many of us facing this stage of life, Maureen has had to reassess who she is without her work to define her and the competitive spirit to drive her. 'I am in that place between being a young woman and an older woman. I have shaken off my career identity and I didn't get to have motherhood as an identity . . . I think that perhaps we all know who we are at the core of us, but historically we have been dressing it up all our lives to fit in. This isn't a negative thing, and I don't feel as if I am in a negative place – quite the opposite. I am excited about the future, but I am changing who I am. I am being kinder to myself, and it is taking some getting used to.

'Now I want to create a mix of doing work I love and [that] intellectually stretches me, with people I like, and spending more time with my family, especially my parents as they age. It's a patchwork of a life I am trying to build, and I don't have all the answers yet, but I feel optimistic and much more confident. I untied myself from the big job because I knew my identity was more than that.'

I sense that the suddenness of Maureen's decision has had a ripple effect that has been lasting for five years already, and the change that has brought in her relationship with herself is what she is dealing with now. She sat in that limbic space, the void between one identity and the next, for just the right amount of time, allowing herself to soften and take the smart decision to move forward into a happier place.

Expect the unexpected

Not all of us can control what the universe throws at us in midlife, though. For some, choice is irrelevant. The week before she turned 50, Jenny was diagnosed with bowel cancer. All her midlife musings suddenly seemed unimportant. Her choices now were limited; her confusion and identity wobbles were all mushed in with the endless chemotherapy and caring for her two teenage children as they dealt with her diagnosis.

'I don't have control over who I am now,' she tells me. 'I am reasonably resilient as a person, I am very much "let's just crack on with it", but this feels like a kick in the teeth, it feels so unfair. I was on one path and suddenly the train shifted tracks. I have no choice now but to deal with it, and it was a shock, it came out of the blue – it is not how I thought life in my fifties would be. I thought by this point I would be invincible because of my life experience.'

Jenny has had to give up work over the past four years to cope with her treatment at the Royal Marsden. She was a chartered surveyor who ran her own business, and her children are in their late teens. As well as having to cope with cancer, she says she is also grappling with feeling aimless without a job. Even when she offered her services to local charities as a volunteer she was turned down.

'No one wants me,' she laughs. 'I feel as if I have no purpose now, which is common among my friends at this age, but mine has another dimension to it because of the cancer. I have no structure to my life. I am from the generation who believed we could have it all. I was the first person in my family to go to university. There was no question of me not working when I had the kids. I just didn't see this coming. We're all in uncharted waters now and it has become a more traditional household with me at home and my husband earning the cash.'

She tells me the cancer has come back in her liver and her lungs. 'This thing has become my job now,' she says. 'It is just non-stop treatment. My actual job came to a halt, and I was such a busy person in my forties. We'd done a lot of travelling with the kids, thank God, and I assumed this tiredness I felt was the usual changes [you'd] expect in midlife.

'But now it is hard to know what was hormones and what was my treatment. "Is it cancer or is it menopause?" I ask myself sometimes. I have lost confidence because of the treatment, but would I have lost it anyway?'

Jenny tells me they were planning her fiftieth birthday party when she found out. It was glorious summer weather, she recalls, but she had a nagging feeling something wasn't right because she was so physically tired (too-tired-to-walk-to-the-car tired).

She didn't tell anyone she'd had a test after a visit to her GP. 'Were you scared?' I asked. 'Scared of being 50? Scared of finding out what was going on?'

'I was just busy,' she says. 'I was more thinking, "How can I lose half a stone by the time of the party on Saturday?" I wasn't scared about being 50 at all; I was confident then, happy about the future. I just wanted to get on with it all and stay busy. Now I am just very sad about it all, particularly when I think of my children and of me not being here for them.

'I want to be around as long as I possibly can, but it is all up in the air right now. The waiting for the results of things is the worst bit. I am a project manager by nature; I just want firm facts and then I can get a plan together, but cancer isn't like that.

'I have to put a brave face on most of the time and protect the children from everything I know about what may or may not happen. I am grabbing as much of this life as we can in between treatments.

'But I don't want life to be a pity party. I don't want this to be all I talk about. I am just cross that in this day and age we haven't found a way to fix this, to stop it happening. I am cross that it is just the luck of the draw.'

151

What Jenny has found in this unexpected twist in her tale is that friendship, particularly the friendship of strong women, has helped her soften her own attitude towards herself.

'I have new women in my life, people who have come to the party with help and love, and I have found some of my friends are much closer to me in a way I had not thought they would be before this diagnosis. I have to accept all the help I am offered now. I think we are prone to a bit of martyrdom and the sense [that] we have to sort everything out as women, and actually I have had to just step back and let people step in for me.'

I say goodbye to Jenny knowing there are no words I can say that will make this situation better for her. I can only feel lucky that I am not in this place myself, and it's a selfish feeling. A week later, by coincidence, I am interviewing a skincare expert in her fifties who was diagnosed with terminal cervical cancer in her early thirties – a woman who was given six months to live, but who now, 20 years later, specialises in aromatherapy. Annee, too, has a quiet sense that you do just have to get on with it, but you also have to find some kindness for yourself along the way when you're dealing with such huge living losses.

What can we learn from women who've faced these big life changes, from those who have had the choices we all seem to be grappling with in midlife taken away from them? Nothing more than the simplest of things: that there is no guarantee of tomorrow, so make today count.

Remember this

Not long after I left the *Sunday Times* we headed home to Cornwall as a family for a summer together. It was the first time we had been able to spend such a long time together.

One afternoon in late summer, I watched quizzically as an ambulance nudged up our tiny lane. Sounds of the beach wafted up the cliff over the house as usual, life carrying on. The ambulance stopped at Tim and Jackie's end-of-lane house for an unusually long while. It left with Jackie, who had died of cancer at home in bed in her late sixties.

Later that month we arranged to visit Tim. We were a few minutes late walking up the lane and met him coming down towards us. 'Can I have a hug, please? I'm missing human company,' he said, the couple's two Labradors walking slowly behind him.

Tim and Jackie had been married for more than 50 years. Jackie was a teacher and Tim a finance director. When they hit their late thirties they moved to Cornwall from Surrey, knowing that one day they wanted to retire here. This sudden but not unexpected (Jackie had been ill for most of that year) ending of their life together felt brutal. It seemed impossible that everything could just continue as it always had and that Tim must continue his life without Jackie. He had opened their small but spectacular garden overlooking the sea for tours – a little poster advertising it sat at the end of the lane, fading in the Cornish sun. He gave any donations to the RNLI. But it wasn't really garden tours he was giving. He would take us around the garden telling the story of Jackie. I think he wanted to keep telling it because he was scared he would forget the specifics of their life and of her.

There was the bench their children bought for her fortieth, the colours she chose, the plants she nurtured. Tim told us the whole story in some detail.

'We met at university,' he said. 'We could hold hands secretly at the back of the lecture theatre and still keep taking notes because I am left-handed and Jackie is right-handed.'

He gave us the tomatoes she grew – the last tomatoes – and a cutting of one of her succulents.

In the front of their garden there was a small decorative fishing boat. A giant flower had grown from a garlic bulb planted in it many years before by one of the couple's children. A name plate on the boat read *Butterdreams*.

'The children called it that,' he remembered. 'I used to sing "Life Is But a Dream" to my daughter at bedtime so we called this boat *Butterdreams*.' His grandchildren were playing around it now.

Tim had lost so much weight I feared for his own health. He talked of carrying on, of his family rallying round and his comforting love of cooking for others, which was keeping him occupied.

The passing of Jackie, who radiated strength and vitality, was quite the wake-up call for all of us. It swiftly brought all our mortalities into view. The end suddenly felt so much nearer. It was a painful reminder of how sleepwalking through the next few years without relishing the new opportunities for change and evolution would be a mistake. Seizing the day was the only course of action now.

10

'Mum, What's the Point of You?'

The morning my eldest was leaving home for university I was violently sick in the downstairs loo. At first I thought it was food poisoning. How bloody unlucky on this day of all days with the long car journey ahead of us. But as a cold film of sweat rippled over my body I realised I wasn't ill at all. I was overwhelmed with sadness. It took over every cell in my body, no matter how hard I tried to override it with logic and stoicism.

As we got ready to leave, the ghost of her as a little girl was still happily racing round our rooms; out of the corner of my eye I still spotted the glitter stubbornly lodged between the floorboards from our days of 'making', strands of her hair on the carpet, her small fingerprints patted onto the grey paint all the way up the stairs, her mugs in the cupboard. It was surprisingly painful, this final letting-go of our first child.

Before I had her I was me, and after her birth my identity changed irrevocably. I was Sky's mum. I have read that cells from your baby stay in your body all your life; your child is forever a physical part of you. They are in your bloodstream, always. Science doesn't know why. But I cling onto that fact every day. It makes me feel a closeness to my children.

In my twenties I didn't think I wanted kids. They weren't part of the plan. My mum had made it sound like hard work and besides, I was ambitious and I loved my job. It was my number-one priority then; I was grateful and sometimes astonished to have achieved what I had.

But I fell in love, and maybe for some of us love changes everything. I was surprised when this maternal longing kicked in shortly after I got married. I'd met James on a blind date five years earlier. He definitely wanted a family, and we were lucky to go on to have four children. Three girls and a boy.

Mothering became a huge part of my identity, not least because alongside editing glossy magazines I wrote a light-hearted weekly newspaper column about it. And then I wrote a book about parenting teenage girls.

Mothering had become intrinsic to who I was. I was as defined by it externally as I was by my job title. I loved being pregnant, loved babies. Even today I love all babies. I was looking forward to motherhood from the day I conceived and immersed myself in the experience. I knew it would shift my identity and I was happy about exploring that. I continued to work full-time after my first, then I did a nine-day fortnight, and finally a four-day week with my fourth child.

There was no question in my mind of giving up a career I'd started at 16, to stay at home with my family. I knew that would be the wrong choice for the type of person I was.

My life was a blend of work, mothering, being part of a couple. Our family unit was a place of constant change; as children grow up we all know the structure of domestic life undergoes relentless rethinking. But for those 18 years we were always parenting four children. It felt as if it consumed us 24 hours a day. It was an intense physical and emotional experience. Choosing to have four children is choosing a busy life, but somehow – even though all mothering is inevitably about this eventual bittersweet separation – I didn't plan for how I would feel on the day that one of them would leave us for good.

Even during that last summer with our eldest still living at home ahead of going to university to study mechanical engineering, I didn't think it would happen. It was a melancholy time, and in the months before departure I seemed to metaphorically polish all the childhood memories of her until they were so clearly visible they sat alongside us making it even sadder. A huge shift in our domestic daily lives and moods occurred in those months, changing us all. Even our Welsh terrier was anxious.

As Pam Ayres writes in her haunting poem about her son leaving home, 'a ghastly leaden feeling like the end of it all' hung over me. A crater appeared and it had happened so quickly and unexpectedly. I mean, I had no idea that one minute we'd be walking to school stopping to check for ladybirds on our front-garden wall, pushing her siblings in a buggy, a trail of raisins behind us, and the very next we would be in Sainsbury's arguing about saucepan quality for shared uni kitchens.

'Shall we take brownies for the other students in the halls on the first day?' I asked her, so needy and desperate for her love and attention I was shamefully trying to please her every minute of every day in the hope that she would realise she was making a terrible mistake and stay at home with me.

'Oh, for God's sake, Lorraine, what's wrong with you?' she replied. 'I'm not going on a playdate. I am not nine.'

I had no idea that the empty peg where her giant puffer coat had hung for many years in our hall would reduce me to tears every time I left the house, no idea that this departure would feel so unexpected and swift, its impact so devastating. I was shocked to the core, we all were.

I had no idea the family dinner on Sunday night without my wonderful daughter's plate at the table would make us cry, that the removal of stuff she liked from the weekly shop would poke this growing bruise of maternal grief.

Of course, I knew about empty nest syndrome; I'd written about it as a journalist and interviewed women who'd written books on it (and it is mostly women). I knew that, yes, the fledglings do boomerang home a lot, yadda yadda yadda, but this loss felt overwhelming, and I was exceptionally unprepared for it. The week before Sky left in September 2020 we were all ill with a minor cold, trying to go about normal life and not think about what was happening, but the anguish was heart-stopping. I am not exaggerating; I had thought all those who used this phrase before about the empty nest were a little OTT until I experienced it myself. So if it is imminent for you, get ready, brace yourself and may the force be with you, because it's brutal, this new form of mourning. Rituals are dismantled, family habits erased, and it all comes without forewarning, having been hiding in plain sight of all parents' eyes. The impact is profound so be prepared, especially if it is your last child leaving or your only child. Your pack is fragmented. You'll never get the band back together again.

You may think, 'What's all the fuss about?' Your kids are meant to go, after all. It's a celebration of a childhood survived and a sign of a thriving future ahead, isn't it? Of parenting well done (most of the time). Your days are now freer, the washing machine is relieved, there are no more trainers clogging up the hall, you know exactly where your tweezers are and the late-night taxi duties are over.

Well, yes to all of that, but it doesn't make up for the end of the golden days (well, they seem more golden in retrospect, that's for sure). This list of 'no mores' – no more holidays governed by term times, no more hardcore rap music or embarrassing encounters with boyfriends or girlfriends in the kitchen – is a good thing and a bad thing, because the other 'no more' list cancels it out. No more nights in watching telly together, no more impromptu card games, no more cuddles on tap, laughter at favourite films, ballgames with the dog, cups of tea in the morning. No more laughing about Dad's hazardous DIY or his list of ailments that grows more comedic each day. Stuff that had a domestic regularity to it is suddenly gone overnight, and that is a visceral feeling of midlife loss.

You are momentarily reduced to a more fragile version of your former maternal self. And usually at this point you are also in the middle of your midlife identity crisis, which is made all the worse when a piece of the jigsaw that has always been there now goes missing. For me, it felt unfair and cruel, especially coming as it did in the middle of the perimenopausal years, and just after Covid and the end of my office job, when I was quickly trying to learn the art of not falling apart completely. We were wrecked as a family by the departure of our capable and kind child, so there seemed little to celebrate about this moment, apart from her being seemingly well prepared (partly by us, we hoped) to go and start this new life.

And that's what you have to keep reminding yourself. One friend tells me she would just say that out loud in the mirror every morning after the last of her three children left: 'I am so pleased for him, he is going to lead such a happy, exciting life.' She said it was a mantra to turn the negative thoughts to optimistic ones – a brain trick.

Every time I opened a cupboard or walked into a room it felt like shelves of Sky's childhood memories were collapsing over me, raining down with happy family scenes. I couldn't go into our lounge without seeing her baby car seat plonked on the carpet the day we first brought her home from hospital and wondered what the hell to do next. I wanted to shout, 'Mind the baby!' every time anyone walked into the room behind me 19 years later.

On the day she left I poured us all tea in the silent gloom of the family morning, a blanket of foreboding huddling us all together. Almost two decades of nostalgia swirled around the cup I was stirring after putting in two sugars. She loves a sweet cup of morning tea. I wasn't ready to say goodbye. I would never be ready. I was even less ready to say goodbye to child number two more than two years later.

Motherhood is, of course, a series of letting-gos; the tide is always going out until the beach is bare and all you see are their little footprints slowly disappearing in the sand.

I felt as though I was dissolving in the face of my eldest's impending absence, pieces of me drifting away as the days passed until she finally had to leave. The morning she left our dog ran around as if searching for some kind of monster lurking in the shadows, her sixth sense alert to the villain of departure.

My husband packed himself a bacon sandwich for the car ride. The other three kids stood solemnly in the kitchen to wave goodbye. Everyone was silent and we were careful not to break any of the teens' obligatory no-touching rules.

I hid my grief and the more extrovert parts of my personality as we dropped her stuff in her new uni room. I watched her say hi to all the new friends she would make, left an I-love-you note in her 'pasta saucepan' (she loves pasta) and bristled a little when she told me she would arrange her room herself and make the bed – a clear statement that none of that kind of mothering was needed now. No speeches, no grand gestures. And then the moment came.

Outside the building we hugged her once (as agreed) and in

the late-September sunshine she turned her back and walked away. Just like that, it was over.

So there you go. If you have children, this is what will happen. The dark shadow of goodbye is hanging over you in midlife. The possibility that you won't be needed as much, and that your value or purpose may therefore be diminished in some way, is one you will have to reckon with. Of course, everyone has a different set-up, a different context for this time of mothering, but for those of you with adolescent children I am asking you not to underestimate the impact of the goodbye. Not to be surprised when your family life, and your relationship with your partner, take on a new dimension, a different way of being. Ignore that at your peril.

I had thought I was wallowing in this moment, or that only a few of us more mentally shaky women were experiencing this pain, but when I went on social media after Sky left I was struck by the number of parents talking about their painful goodbyes, all of us in shock, as if we were sharing an unspeakable secret. Why had these feelings come as such a surprise?

It comes after a summer when you don't see your teens much at all. This is the vanishing summer, the one after the stress of exams when they suddenly take to the road with their mates, only popping back home to leave a few towels all over the bathroom floor and tell you that your 'breathing is too loud'.

I asked those with older children if I was overreacting and they said no. I asked my parents and they agreed it was terrible, awful. I don't think there is a cure for empty-nest agony; it's like jumping into what you think will be a hot bath but finding out the water is actually freezing cold. If you know these feelings are coming then perhaps the experience is less scary. You can plan to occupy yourself: get a hobby, redecorate, find those new friends, change the routine, travel – anything to distract you for a moment before you feel the loss, because feeling the loss is important. Be sensitive to your teens before they go; ease off on complaining about the dirty laundry and mucky cups under the bed for this last part of your parenting ride, because they won't be there for long.

Living with teens

It's a tumultuous family time, this domestic midlife messiness, because it comes straight after that other rite of passage: your descent into the most annoying superhero of all: 'Moron Mum'. This happens gradually as your children turn into teens and start viewing you as the idiot they live with. Often they stop calling you Mum and use your first name instead, or they make one up, like my son calling me Morag.

It seems to me they start to discard your mothering role ahead of time. It's illogical, I know, but I found being called Lorraine by my girls as irritating as listening to the relentless chorus of 'Mum, Mum, Mum' at times when they were little, a chorus that had been my soundtrack up until this point. It was upsetting; I wasn't ready to not be Mum.

Obviously the huge changes in the teenage brain that occur during adolescence are the reason for this (I wrote a whole book about not taking it personally), but a furious perimenopausal woman who can't remember which side of the road to drive on, living with a 'meanager' who consistently undermines everything about her, is a shadow of her former self by the time she gets to the uni drop-off.

The timing of all this is the worst aspect for many of us. Don't get me wrong, I love everything about teens, especially my teens, who I'd step in front of a runaway train for, but all the developmental stages they go through as they mature seem to clash with the ones many of us face as we're in the middle of an identity crisis. It's the perfect hormonal storm and no one has any patience, especially if you have girls.

They steal your stuff from your bathroom and deny it with such authority that you feel like you are going mad, or they accuse you of 'ruining' their lives if you ask for it back.

If you're occasionally feeling brave, you end up taking petty revenge on them: Marmite on the butter knife is a good one. ('What's wrong with you, Mum? How can you live with yourself?' is what they will say if you do that.)

They set your Netflix profile to Jabba the Hutt for a laugh (obviously, you have no idea how to correct this. You don't even know the Netflix password anymore).

They'll dismiss all your endeavours with 'she's doing some swimming/running/writing thing' and question all your career choices as their hormones run wild and they separate from you in what feels like the most painful way possible.

In our house I would be hiding all the small things my teen daughters were 'borrowing' and forever forgetting where they were, then getting cross about having to hide them in the first place. We could open a corner shop selling tweezers, good scissors, new trainer socks and all the 'good' mascaras if we could find the ones I'd squirrelled away.

My two eldest would frequently and carelessly ask, 'What's the point of you?' after some of our rows, and for a while the Armageddon-like menstrual periods that we all seemed to have at the same time saw the trio of us walking around guzzling iron supplements like addicts. And for me, it was also a little dispiriting to see their soft, unlined, much-loved skin every day after I'd looked in the mirror at my own not-so-lovable wrinkles. They looked normal, and I looked like I was wearing an 'old suit'. They were there accidentally reminding me of the past I missed, that other beginning I had already been through in my own teens that I would never experience again. And one of our girls looked so uncannily like me as a teen that my dad said he did a heart-stopping double-take every time he saw her.

The house was full of hormones – the abundance of theirs and the fluctuating decrease of mine. We were all going through some form of synchronised identity crisis; the difference was, they were building theirs and I was losing little bits of mine. Plus, I had to be there for the one they were experiencing. I was on duty, shepherding them through it, in between misplacing my belongings, grappling with my own swirly octopus of emotions and standing in a cold shower each morning pushing a lid down on the inexplicable rage. Up until this point, I noted, parenting had been a little easier, but now I was expected to be much more skilled. This was the time for *Top Gun* parenting, for the elite of the elite, and yet I often felt I was growing evermore rubbish as a mum. One or other of my children would want to talk to me urgently late at night when I was at my most useless. By 8.30 p.m. I barely knew my surname, but I would have to sit up in bed or chat in the dark with a teen experiencing overwhelming emotions, some that she was struggling to handle. Listening is such a hard skill when you are perpetually confused and overwhelmed by life yourself. But listen you must.

I knew my eldest two girls needed to simultaneously cling to me and push me away in their quest for independence; this is hard to take when you're clinging onto your own sanity and pushing away the parts of you that don't serve you well anymore. It's especially hard when you are setting new boundaries around what you feel you can do well for others. And it's even harder when you are also caring for elderly parents. Friends of mine were mothering teens and their elderly mums too – it can be overwhelming if you don't ask for help or show how vulnerable all this makes you feel. So, if you are in this situation right now, acknowledge that all this is going on and that it is difficult to deal with. You won't get it right all the time, so give yourself a break every now and again.

Mothering: How did I do?

Just before I got to the uni drop-off, I had started to be ambushed by uncomfortable motherhood memories, the wake-you-up-in-the-night worries where I came to believe, in my midlife madness, that I had done it all wrong – messed up this blend between work and mothering. Should I have left them when they were little? Should I have given up working full-time? Should I have had fewer children? Was I attentive enough? Did I shout too much? Should I have been writing about them in a national newspaper as I did on a weekly basis? There were so many questions I worried I had been too distracted to answer before.

This questioning is yet another surprise revelation that will make you feel as if you are going mad.

I was in the position of having four children a decade apart, my first at 33 and my last at 43. I'd had a baby at the beginning of my editing career and a baby in the midst of one of my successful periods of work, where I had more power to ask for what I wanted (and the experience of working motherhood to know what I realistically needed in order to get everything done to serve everyone well). Mine was the main salary for our family, and I had invested a huge chunk of my life in my career from the age of 16. I wasn't prepared to step out, so I did both: work and motherhood. But at what cost?

Obviously the context here is particular to me: like many Londoners, we had no parental help because both sets of grand-parents lived hundreds of miles away, but we were able to afford paid-for childcare as working parents. I had a degree of

165

flexibility in my work; I had gone in my job from the country to the city, from no qualifications to winning awards for journalism. And I'd chosen to have four children. All of it was my choice: my choice to work and parent, to live in a city, to have a large family and a dog, to be married. As I talk about in Chapter 5, I'm of the generation of women who felt we had to 'have it all' and not complain, not examine the dark corners of it. And now I felt I had to keep quiet about this creeping sense of doubt over my role as a mother that had slipped into my midlife mind.

Alongside 'keeping mum' about the sheer scale of stuff to remember and do as a working mother when I first started my family, the concept of motherhood as a vocation was snowballing in society during my editorship of *Cosmopolitan* in 2002.

Motherhood, rather than mothering, had apparently become some kind of near-religious experience then, its cultural value growing rapidly, and at that point in the late nineties and early noughties you kind of had to roll up your sleeves and embrace the child-centred motherhood diktats of the growing cult of 'motherphilia'. The notion of attachment parenting – having a constant physical and emotional closeness to your baby – was becoming mainstream. If you worked out of the home you'd have to pump breast milk in the loo before going to a board meeting (which I often did) and then come home, whip off your blouse and have skin-to-skin time with your little one. I felt I was being asked to be all things to everyone all the time in a way that my husband was not.

Motherhood was judged at every turn, whether you were a biological mum or not, a so-called stay-at-home mum or a working mum, and there were so many silent expectations around it when I first had kids. Every time any of us walked out of the door as mums all eyes were on us, and we were flooded with unsolicited advice on how to do it under this new cult of motherphilia. It was an odd experience: the mothering was joyous, but the motherhood stressful. All of this stuff romped through my head in the sweaty perimenopausal nights as my teens headed towards their eventual departure. Did I do it right?

In a world where we were paid less than men and in every respected statistical survey ever done we came off worse in terms of health and happiness, there were still so many expectations around working women. Like most of them, at the time I went with the flow – it was my choice – but really I should have stepped out of the river, stood on the bank and thought about what was actually going on in society. Women were being expected to do so much without flexibility in the workplace to support them, without support for the mental load at home. Some working women questioned this but many of us just carried on. Perhaps our millennial sisters are more vigilant. I hope so.

I didn't anticipate this retrospective worry and throwback shame around parenting. I was of course overthinking everything, which was not a habit of mine up until this messy midpoint. I kept remembering the Sunday when I had to stop feeding one of my babies to go back to work on the Monday; it horrified me in the early hours when at the time it had seemed my only option, heart-breaking as it was.

Of course, in the sensible daylight hours I had none of these doubts. I didn't attribute any problems I'd encountered in my parenting to me working. I knew I had missed moments of my kids' childhoods, but pre-midlife me was fine with that. And mums who worked from home or didn't work at all no doubt had just as many worries about their parenting as those who worked outside of the home.

I truly loved my work, and I loved mothering too, so I am not grumbling or being defensive here, or indeed judging any other woman's choices. Nonetheless, when I look at the columns

I wrote in early motherhood I can see that I *was* extremely defensive about my choices then – fighting back against the criticism, I suppose – which of course I regret now. I don't, however, regret the decisions I made. And I don't feel guilty, because guilt implies doing something wrong, which is not what working mothers do – they have committed no crime. Perhaps we didn't take time out to think about how we could have had an easier time – an experience that is more open now, I hope, to younger women. But we probably never took time out to congratulate ourselves on the times we got things right for ourselves and our families either.

A fellow mum my age tells me her children always began a conversation with her with 'I know you are busy, but can I just . . .' Now she shudders remembering that. 'How could I have been too busy to talk to my kids?' she thinks. We all have those thoughts, but I think if we can notice them and let them go, we won't default to the Gen-X mindset of 'I should have been better at this', or the daft idea that there are rules for mothering the right way – there aren't.

Mothering or not mothering: a midlife reckoning

Women without children at this stage of their lives have told me of a different kind of landmine exploding as they grappled with their midlife identity.

I spoke to one woman, now in her early fifties, who had not been able to conceive for many years and when she did she had several miscarriages, which she thinks led to the breakdown of her relationship.

'I realise I have been through a living loss with my miscarriages,' she told me. 'I need to mourn that rather than keep pushing on. If I look back I now wonder, if I had been kinder, more compassionate to myself, would I have not had the miscarriages? Did I do something wrong to not get pregnant?'

No matter what the circumstances, our generation's tendency seems to be to blame ourselves. And while trying to find peace with her pregnancy losses, at the same time, like all of us, this woman has been negotiating a major midlife identity shift. 'I've met someone new and we know we won't be able to have children now,' she explained. 'Which is hard to come to terms with as I age. But I have just decided to get softer with age, to be less hard on myself at work and about achieving . . . I have stepped out of a big career and started to study again. I am slowing down and creating space for my new identity. It is hard, but I think it is a better way to be.'

As we chatted we considered the word 'restless'; perhaps as Gen-X working women we had been so driven we now found it hard to be less focused in these years. Maybe this was why we were all finding this stage of life so tricky to deal with. It required a skill we didn't have as a generation.

'I feel like I may be finding the core of who I am now, that for years I dressed it up as this fierce working woman, which may not be who I really am,' she agreed.

My childless friend also talked of feeling lonely without the children she thought she would have, and she feels for her younger self when perhaps she didn't acknowledge her loneliness, which often appeared in the form of anxiety.

The loss of the chance at motherhood for those who want it is no doubt felt keenly by women at this stage of life, because of course this is one of the things you won't get a second chance at.

I also spoke to a single mum who had had a child at 37 with donor sperm after 'being very bad at relationships with men', as she told me. She ran her own career-coaching business and seemed to be working doubly hard as both Mum and Dad alongside her career.

'I have been holding it together as a single woman ever since I got pregnant,' she explained (she is now in her early fifties). 'I am now a mum and also a daughter to ageing parents who need help, and it feels like there is little space for me in this place. I am hoping I make my fifties mean something, that I don't want to 'just get through it'.

'There are a lot of women like me as mums – we don't often hear their stories, though. I had to ask for help a lot as a single mother, even with paid-for childcare, so I learned what that felt like, which I think is useful to me now during this questioning phase of life. It is useful to be able to ask for help in midlife.'

She told me she had had to adapt her Gen-X coping mindset because single parenting is doubly demanding in our rigid, inflexible society; 'enduring' your mothering alone does not work; you often need to soften and ask for the support of others simply to get through your day if you work.

And she also told me that the story of why she is single is one of the trickiest parts of the experience, because most people expect her to explain that her child's father left, rather than the fact that she made a choice not to have a father in her daughter's life.

'People assume that I had an accidental baby, or that there is a tragic story of a man leaving or dying. It feels convenient to have the idea of a man leaving us, to others, but I have always been honest about why I am a single mum and sometimes society finds that confusing. We don't like to think women can be so proactive in their choices around motherhood,' she explained.

It is perhaps even harder for her to define an identity in midlife when most women are expected to be in a relationship at this stage. The traditional narrative of family life and how it is supposed to be by the midpoint is so strong, I wonder if she feels any sense of failure around her situation? Refreshingly, she does not.

'I feel a little lost sometimes,' she says. 'And my identity is perplexing because I am not my younger self, though I feel a huge urge to get back in touch with her now my daughter is older . . . There is a huge simplicity in doing things alone. I do still have to deal with stress and the need for a sense of achievement, but I love my work right now. I have a sense of energy and I am not looking for another person in my life to make it complete.'

Who mothered you?

Changing your perspective as the demands of motherhood lessen (to an extent – I am still booking my eldest's haircuts!) perhaps offers a rare moment to embrace new thinking. This is something I discovered when I interviewed the author Tanya Shadrick for the podcast. She wrote *The Cure for Sleep: Memoir of a Late-waking Life*, a book about her near-death experience, after her first child was born, from a blood clot. It beautifully describes how some women struggle with the concept of motherhood in the way we live it today, and she also tackles her affair in her early forties when she tried, but failed, to be in love with two men and live a life with both of them.

It's an extraordinary book and Tanya offers so many thoughtful perspectives on taking the road less travelled. It's an exploration of 'getting free of the opinion of others, living outside of what was normal in my time and place'. I was particularly struck by her idea of beginning a transformation to a new way of living by writing a list of what you love – 100 things. She told us that as soon as women got to around 60 or so, the list became very personal and one really started to get a picture of what life could be next – the start of a creative journey. It's around the 60 mark that you have to dig deep and admit the things you really need.

I thought creating this list would be a good thing for midlife women to do as the chains of motherhood loosened, as the sacrifices made were acknowledged but now put aside for us to find something more for ourselves – a shift in our identity defined by a list of things that brought us great joy. Tanya's book is a pathfinder for midlife women even though it isn't about that. It is also a bit about rule breaking, which is something we are probably more in the mood for after the age of 45. After all, midlife can be a time to experiment and play, to risk making a contrary decision or taking a path you have so far avoided, perhaps because the chores of motherhood have restricted you.

Notwithstanding the heartache of empty nest syndrome, it is good to acknowledge that it can be a positive to be released from the compelling and constricting agendas around motherhood. For some, it may feel like moving from constantly coping to finally living. It is a time to step forward into a new kind of liberation, a freedom from responsibilities. Many women I've spoken to have also chosen this freedom by stepping away from relationships and marriages – those who stayed in them (rightly or wrongly) 'for the children'.

Plans without family can now be made. Indeed, many of the mums in our midlife podcast community have worked through the grief of losing their mothering roles and come out the other side with plans for new beginnings. They had the extra time filled already.

I am now learning to let those critical thoughts I have around my own mothering pop up and pass through, like trains moving through a station, without judging them or even answering the questions. I know they will still come, but now I watch them sail by, rather than letting the shame descend. I look at my own mother and grandmother, and see what I may or may not have inherited in the making of my own identity.

Thinking all this through prompted me to complete the genogram exercise (which therapists often recommend for personal development and self-awareness). This is where you spend a few hours plotting the pathways of your family tree as far back as you can, describing those relatives in detail and their way of connecting or being.

I noticed that on the genogram map of my past, the overriding pattern in my family was a distance from each other, both emotional and physical. I had not broken that pattern by coming so far away from home so early on, I realised; in fact, quite the opposite. It was also true that nothing was ever discussed out loud in my family; letters were written instead, significant happenings were left undiscussed, important feelings were buried, in my opinion – a common trait of the boomer generation before us. The outside world seemed to be something to fear in many pockets of the family I am from, and very little is known about our ancestry beyond my grandparents. We're not talkers or sharers; the connections are not strong. Now that I can see this drawn out in black and white, I want to avoid it with my four children and the family I have pulled around them from my husband's side (the distance doesn't exist there).

I highly recommend you try creating your own genogram (see page 236 for books that can help you), because it highlights patterns you may want to encourage or avoid in your own relationships as you work through the midlife identity crisis. Family is, after all, where your identity began.

This quest to find out who we are as we age is complicated after the motherhood years, isn't it? Navigating the new dynamics of your relationship if you are in one; finding value and purpose again as your internal landscape changes. Obviously you are still mothering, and then possibly grandmothering, but when the up-to-your-knees-in-it, swirly phase ends as we age, the world of family life is so very different.

Only one of my four kids calls me Mum now, and she's on the cusp of rejecting that description. I remember when I had her, the gynaecologist offered to 'sterilise' me during the planned C-section. It would be simple and take no more than a few seconds. I was almost 44, it made sense, but I said no.

It was a visceral reaction – I said no immediately. Whether it is wise to ask a heavily pregnant woman this question in the first place, I don't know, but deep inside I felt that if I said yes, it would completely alter my identity. It was mad and illogical, but I didn't want to lose the absolute proof that I was a mother the day I gave birth. Of course, when you go through the menopause and your ovaries stop working, *that* is the final proof you won't ever be a biological mother again, but once you have had children, nothing can take away the fact that you *are* a mother.

What I have learned now is that, even though it will always be part of you, motherhood is indeed a constant letting-go, not just of your children, but gradually of your mothering. In midlife you let go of many parts of yourself, and you may need to shake off that intense maternal part of you like a dog shaking off sand after a run on the beach. This will be good for you in the long run – holding on to it weighs you down. As mothers we all feel as if we have been forged in fire – all those years of maternal toil have given us strength and purpose. Maybe we can divert some of that energy into mothering ourselves now.

11

Turning the Light on in the Fridge: A Peek into the Future

By this point you should feel better prepared for this messy middle bit of life, these transformations, the losses large and small, the constant changes ahead. You know what 'liminal' means (see page 88), you're less of a hot mess, and when you point at the TV remote and say, 'Pass me the thing that changes the picture on the thing on the wall,' you know it's just a momentary dip in your 'smarts' and not the end of days. There's nothing wrong with you and you are not going mad. All the stuff mentioned in the previous chapters is 'relatable' and you should hopefully feel less alone. Perhaps a self-management plan is forming. Perhaps the softening has begun and maybe you are beginning to savour all these changes, rather than force your way through some sort of reinvention.

But what news from the advance party? The women further ahead of us on this road? They've already gone through passport control and boarded the plane – what can they tell us about the upsides of this so-called second spring? The female midlife experience has been ignored for so long that we haven't heard as many positive stories as we should have from those who have gone through it already. Our podcast, *Postcards from Midlife*, was the first to specifically look at all aspects of female midlife, and our community grew swiftly because the thirst for this kind of information, these kinds of stories, is snowballing. Women of our age want to feel part of something and to belong, and we want to be prepared.

The good news is that older women have many uplifting stories to tell. I have loved listening to them when we've interviewed them on the podcast and when I chatted to them for this book. They were keenly aware that it is our attitudes that shape our futures. It will be our decision on whether to be positive or negative about ageing that will define us the most.

When we asked older women about their experiences they told powerful tales of a new equilibrium, of happiness, acceptance, tranquillity, sanity regained. I felt so lucky to learn that these uncomfortable feelings, these issues we experience, are usually temporary (although, of course, there are no absolutes here).

As we've discussed, preparation is key to reaching this state. Knowing that these feelings are coming your way as you head into your mid-forties does prepare you for them, and it means you can start to think about how you'll handle it and perhaps develop some coping strategies. If you aren't ambushed by it then it won't feel so terrifying and you won't temporarily lose sight of yourself, as many of us have done. If you can make sense of where you are, then you can make the best possible decisions about what happens next. You won't feel as if something is wrong with you.

The element of surprise that women experience, and their consequent lack of preparation, seems to be what differentiates the sexes when it comes to the so-called 'midlife crisis' years. For men, dissatisfaction appears to be the main issue; they don't seem, from my research, to feel so ambushed by it all. Culturally, there is more talk of their coming 'midlife crisis', which doubtless helps them prepare for it. And, of course, it's easier for them in other ways too, because their biological clock ticks so much more slowly than ours, and society ages them more gradually as a result – leading men in films, for example, still date or marry women way younger than them. But for women it is the shock, rather than feeling cheated, that dominates their experience, which is why the lessons we've learned from the older women we've talked to were so heartening. They just wanted to step through the right doorways to their future life, to find peace but also excitement, to be reinvigorated and to feel valued. It's a manifesto at odds with what is being sold to us in Western society, though.

In many other parts of the world the story is very different. In Mayan culture, older women are seen as wiser, as leaders; they are revered. In Japan there is a respect for post-menopausal women that we don't experience here, and it seems to be reflected in their health, with women there reporting fewer physical symptoms of perimenopause and menopause. A more positive attitude to ageing seems to imply a less problematic transition. Women in Native American cultures and in Papua New Guinea also enjoy an increased social standing as they age.

This positivity is something to embrace, but we need to seek it out; it doesn't happen in our culture because we're still labouring under Freud's disputed idea that motherhood is a woman's sole purpose and that when that ends we are of less value. This idea has suited the patriarchy for so long, in my opinion, that it's hard to see how we can change it, but by talking about these new positive attitudes we can hopefully pass them around among women. And with more and more women getting into positions of power and influence, they can start to make the structural changes that will benefit us all. Personally,

177

I have decided that even if our Western world doesn't confer the status of elder, wiser woman upon me, I will happily apply it to myself.

So hearing older women's stories is incredibly important in helping us navigate our way through midlife to the wisdom beyond. They're nourishing, they're motivating, and the dearth of them in our culture has been a disgrace, which is why I decided to write this book.

Many of our guests on *Postcards from Midlife* spoke of hitting an emotional loneliness in their mid and late forties, and, if that's how you feel, it's vital to know that you are not alone, even if it seems that way. Therapist and parenting guru Philippa Perry, who is in her sixties, came on the show and told us how much better we would all feel if we were given advance notice of this midlife crisis. Perry, who says her main symptom of perimenopause before HRT was 'wanting to murder everyone', explained how women go from alpha to beta during midlife. It's this change that causes much of the confusion, she thinks.

'As alpha adults we're gathering resources, and when we turn into beta adults we're starting to enjoy the resources, so alpha-adult-you buys the allotment and beta-adult-you likes to dig the garden. Now, unless anyone tells us we are going from alpha to beta, it isn't surprising we feel strange and discombobulated. So I advise you to ask yourself in this time of life: "What am I feeling now? What do I want to do now? What's right for me now?" Then you can go for it. We can keep an eye on the death maths, acknowledge we are sad [that] we know we will die one day, but keep moving on all the same.'

Forewarned is forearmed, and moving forward, as Philippa recommends, is surely the healthiest response. This is why, personally, I don't like all the messages we get about 'resisting' growing older that society gives us. This just makes the confusion around what is going on for us even worse. I'm not saying that one morning you will wake up having forgotten all the words to Duran Duran's 'Rio' and craving a carvery for tea at 6 p.m. – accepting ageing is not about giving up and putting your slippers on – I am saying try not to get drawn into thinking that attempting to recapture your youth is resistance. It isn't; to me it feels like denial and a refusal to see the opportunities ahead. And you don't want to miss those.

Time for some PMA (positive mental attitude)

This new stage of life comes with many positives. One of my favourites is the ability to be who you are without worrying what people around you think. And being more confident about saying no is a gift. I stole the phrase 'That sounds like a you problem' from my teenagers and it has become an increasingly useful response at times when I don't want to step in and sort things out for everyone else: when I want to say no.

Learning not to do things that will overwhelm you is powerful too; doing it all is not ideal for young or old. As Philippa Perry told us, 'Women are so used to having so many plates spinning. All these roles, all these hats they wear . . . but what about you? You need that me-time; if you don't have it, you get exhausted and your mind cranks up that critical voice in your head. Those illogical criticisms come up – the "I can't drive any more", "I can't do my job", "I am a bad mother" – so you need to stop and rest. This voice isn't really saying, "You can't do this"; it is really saying, "Please slow down."'

This slowing-down as we age, of doing less but doing it well, is a liberation for many of us; it is our permission to live a less stressful life. Reframing your mindset around all the things you have in your life is a powerful exercise. And even if you cannot change difficult circumstances, you can change your attitude to them. I think we sometimes get used to believing we are too busy to say no. We overwhelm ourselves because it is familiar and therefore feels safer than not being overwhelmed. But there are many small 'nos' that even the busiest of us, those who may have no choice around our daily responsibilities, can say. As Philippa explained to us, 'Our bodies are different at this stage, and we need to take time to get to know ourselves again. We need more time with our peers. And we should try and arrange our lives to accommodate our need for a slower pace.'

You may find you become more patient as you age, which is helpful and takes the lid off the stress pot. You'll probably enjoy the lack of monthly periods after menopause, as well as the release from all the premenstrual chaos you may have endured in the past. Many midlife women stop overthinking too; they accept that they may get it wrong sometimes, and that it is OK. Women told us they became more playful in later life as they relaxed their attitudes towards themselves. And you can save a bit of the rage that comes in around 45 for the times when you want to stand up for yourself, the times when you have decided you are too old to bend around others, when you complain about something or ask for exactly what you need.

I can, of course, see how even the word 'positivity' (coming as it does from the dictionary of wellness waffle) might set off the eye-rolling among the more cynical of us, trapped in our traditional way of being, but if you suffer from this resistance to self-care stuff because it feels like it doesn't belong in your world, trust me, it won't be helpful for you now. Midlife is a time to drop the prejudice around previously held ideas, to be open-minded and not dismiss the things older women from beyond your world are saying.

Be more curious. Soften yourself. And be prepared to know that what you held to be true before may not be true now. Change is constant and you can't hide from that. Don't be afraid to be seen as the person you may have been covering up all these years with all those steel-trap coping strategies. Vulnerability is a helpful midlife tool, as we have established. It's likeable. So adapt and evolve.

In my case, I realised this 'strong' cynical mindset was keeping everyone at a distance, but the softer version of me doesn't have to do that anymore. I've learned that letting people in isn't dangerous or weak. On the contrary, keeping everyone at a distance may make you feel lonelier as you age. Perhaps it comes out of a fear that if people get close and see who you really are, they may not like you, but taking a step back and reviewing that is worth trying, because we can change.

My yoga teacher, Nadia Narain, a new friend I made in my late forties, says she watched me shift from that closed person to a more vulnerable, open woman. Obviously, coming from my background, even typing 'yoga teacher' makes me cringe, but I have started to ignore that inner voice telling me that people like me don't do yoga or practise self-care, because it is unhelpful and illogical.

When I met Nadia her life was in transition too, so much so that we had her on the show to talk about finding love in her late forties, a love for which she chose to give up a full-time career, with a 30-year legacy behind it, and move to the US to be with her new boyfriend and his family of two teenagers. It was an extraordinary change for her, out of the blue and utterly unexpected.

'As I got older,' she told us on the show, 'I realised that I didn't want any drama in my life. I didn't want to start drama or be part of drama. I wanted just nice, calm relationships. I grew up in full-blown drama and got to this point in life after being addicted to it. I would gravitate towards it; the more drama, the more in love I was, but in my early forties I made a decision to stop it.

'It does not serve me anymore. I can walk away from it. I felt like I needed to take control again as I aged.'

This ability to walk away from drama is a good tip for the transition stage. Nadia also brought us the best piece of midlife advice, which I urge all Gen-X women to take on board, because it has certainly worked for me.

'"Stay soft, not strong" is a great mantra for midlife women,' she said. 'Be honest, be vulnerable, ask for help.'

When TV presenter Kate Garraway came on the show, she also talked about letting go of the ideas around who you are as you age. She arrived in our studio shortly after coming out of *I'm a Celebrity . . . Get Me Out of Here* in the Australian jungle. I marvelled at the idea that this incredibly introverted woman had felt able to go to the other side of the world, minus her family, and appear on live TV in a bikini, aged 49.

'I found myself thinking that when I turned 50 it could be a gentle glide to wonderfulness,' she told us. 'But in the jungle I found a strange thing. I actually realised I'd always been seeking the easiest possible option in life, but if you only seek comfort, you begin to lose the thrill of the world opening up, like you had in your twenties.

'We have a story we tell ourselves, that we are "that" sort of person, and it becomes who we are, but it doesn't have to be. I am a scared person, but I did more than I thought I would in the jungle. Then you start thinking, "Well, I can do these things" [and] life becomes more of a choice and less of a closing-down. New things come to you, and midlife is about resetting your life in the direction you want, rather than decreasing the circles.'

I loved this take on midlife, this expansive attitude, the positivity behind it, but it requires us to come to terms with the idea that our core values might change and to deal with all the losses that nibble away at us as we age – the living losses that therapist Julia Samuel, now into her sixties, talked about when she came on the podcast to answer listeners' questions.

I loved having Julia on the show, because her advice was so specific and practical; she advocates seeing the positive in acknowledging the sense of loss we may feel in midlife, whether or not we are actually grieving for something or someone. It's advice that applies to us all, as that feeling of loss seems to bleed across all women's experiences.

She said it all comes down to the quality of our relationships; it is this that dictates how positively we go forward into the future because we live or die by those connections, and we crave love and attention as humans. She reinforced this idea I had noticed cropping up on WhatsApp: that we may become invisible, feel ignored and perhaps feel exiled from our tribe because we've grown older and our lives are so different from how they were. We're not mums of young children anymore, some of our offspring have left, our bodies have changed, our jobs have changed; we've moved into an uncomfortable place in many cases. This discomfort of not being who I used to be was one of the things that really troubled me, but the discomfort is the important bit – you can't ignore it.

'Many of the people I counsel have a clock in their head of where they [think they] should [be] by their mid-forties,' Julia told us. 'And if they [haven't done] what they planned they would then they feel as if they sleepwalked into their forties and then woke up and missed all opportunities, leaving them facing a brick wall, a dark, frightening future.

'So it may be helpful to think about reframing this feeling and envisage a future with hope. Hope is the alchemy of change, but it means you have to have the courage to face yourself in midlife. And pain is an agent of change; it tells us to wake up because something is not right; if you block this pain, the more stuck you are in a place of discomfort and the louder the signals will get. They are there to protect us and shift our lens. You have to face up to that and feel liberated to be yourself, to see all of you, to be vulnerable, show yourself.'

It gets better and better

The women in their early sixties who came on the show shone a light on the 'what next?' question for us. They all had the same upbeat mindset. It was lightbulb moment after lightbulb moment as we heard their stories. For me, they closed the gap between what had sometimes felt like the worst of times and what could, according to them, be the best of times in the future, and they preached an easier acceptance of 'the worst' when it happened. This was the next stop on the tube line for us and it reinforced the idea that once you are out of the void, it would all be OK.

We had not set out to interview women who were technically no longer in midlife for our podcast, but we did realise early on that those women had been largely ignored by the media until now – we had not heard, watched or read their wisdom before, but we knew we needed that wisdom to be captured to spur us on. In my head, the idea of turning 60 had always felt like the end of the world as we know it; it is, after all, a largely unexplored female landscape. But 60 becomes a beacon for some women, especially those who have had a close female relative die before that age.

Patsy Kensit, whose mum died of cancer at 53, told us she was looking forward to the liberation of turning 60. An icon in the '80s and '90s whose whole persona was tied to being a symbol of youthful adventures, Patsy was overjoyed about the possibility of 'making it' to 60.

The stories we heard from women already in their seventh decade removed the element of foreboding that I had initially felt when we started the podcast in 2020. At that point, I felt stranded in midlife, as if I was the only one feeling the weight of the death maths, the horror of time running out. But the more we talked to women who were already in what seemed like that far-away future, the more I realised none of us is marooned alone in our ages. There are women in front of us and around us able to offer up good news, inspiration and comforting reassurance. Hallelujah to them.

The author Kate Mosse told us she thought her fifties felt to some extent like a continuation of her forties but that 60 was a very different world to be in – something exciting and new. She has written much about being with her elderly parents in their dying hours, and that experience, she told us, led her to wonder what her story will be when the end comes, but also to realise that you can take more chances as you age. 'Leap and the net will find you,' she advised.

I felt incredibly optimistic after spending time with Kate, because everything 'big' in terms of success and family had happened to her in her forties and fifties – as it had for many women we interviewed – and yet she believed her sixties would be even better. She had such youthful hope and positivity, which felt sensible and logical, not a fantasy that hid a fear of death or ageing.

Talking to these wise elders brought smiles to our faces and reinforced what we do of course all know deep down already: that being thinner, being richer, being more popular and having more stuff doesn't make you happy. Of the many women over 60 I interviewed, almost without exception they had all embraced being grateful for the lives they were leading and talked of 'finding themselves' as they aged.

One of my favourite interviews for this book was with an

American woman in her eighties, who had seen much tragedy but also much happiness in her life – or rather lives.

'I am 84 and every day is gosh darn exciting,' she told me. Judy Glickman Lauder has four children and 16 grandchildren. She was married to her first husband Albert for 54 years until he died in 2013. Then two years later she married one of their best friends, Leonard Lauder, also a widower, chairman emeritus of The Estée Lauder Companies. Leonard had been married to his late wife Evelyn for 52 years until her death from ovarian cancer in 2011. Judy and Leonard were married by two of Judy's sons and one of her daughters-in-law, who are all rabbis.

I had sat next to Judy at a beauty-industry lunch four years before we spoke for this book. At that point in my life I was in the eye of the storm of midlife. Confused, increasingly fatigued, discombobulated and wondering what was going on inside my soul. And then one day there was Judy, offering a glimpse of sunlit possibilities in the tomorrows ahead of me. I found her quite incredible. There was a sense of peace around her that was intoxicating for a woman living in the middle of chaos as I was.

Judy is a photographer whose work has included chronicling the Holocaust death camps, a project paying respect to her European background. She has seen great loss, been through much herself, but she is also living a wonderful life with her new husband. They described themselves as romantic with a capital R, and the giddiness between them was quite something to watch given that they had known each other for decades already. I stayed in touch with Judy after we first met and commissioned a piece on her later-life romance for *Sunday Times Style*. I was intrigued by her sense of peace and really looking for the doorway that led to it myself.

'How does it feel looking back at your forties and fifties now?' I asked.

'I never imagined then I would start so many new lives,' she laughs as we chat on the phone post-pandemic. 'The most important thing I have learned is to be grateful for everything, at each age and stage. It's been the most-used word of my life.'

She tells me that in her fifties she was overcome with an urge to step outside of her day-to-day life; she wanted to travel, to go to India.

'I'd never really travelled by myself. I was immersed in family and work up until then and I just wanted to experience this alone. I had reached an age where I decided I could give myself permission to do things, even though everyone told me not to. I think that's what you get in midlife, a sense of giving yourself permission to explore.

'I landed in Bombay at 3 a.m., alone. It was a big break from everything I was doing at home. And you know, that's my advice for younger women: always leave the door open for something completely different, make room to plant new seeds.'

I am aware that Judy leads a more privileged life than most, but I quote her because what she says is what all the older women told me, whatever their background. Judy herself has observed that privilege doesn't necessarily solve things. 'You know, in the world I mix in,' she says, 'I know a lot of people who have everything they want in life, everything, and yet they are still unhappy. As life happens you must always be grateful for every chance that pops up.'

Her outlook resonates with all the coaching and counselling experts I have interviewed. This sense of mortality, which quietly tugs on our sleeves as we head into our fifties, has a deeper bite at Judy's age. At her age, she tells me, you lose people every day. 'It really takes it out of you, those phone calls,' she adds.

Before I hang up on our chat, she tells me: 'Life is a little sprinkle of everything. I see each morning as a new beginning. Every age we reach has new rewards, so focus on them.'

And that seems to be the source of her peace. Another woman in her seventies – stylish, single, travelling the world alone, living new lives – told me she has chosen to be 'surprised and curious about all the changes rather than disappointed or fearful', even in the face of trauma (her husband died of a heart attack beside her in his fifties). I found this perfectly logical idea of choosing your mindset incredibly helpful. Even my cynical brain likes looking for the upside in dire situations.

When I was editing *Sunday Times Style* I signed food writer Nigella Lawson as a columnist; she was in her late fifties at the time. We would chat weekly on the phone about future subjects, and I once spent a lovely afternoon with her (she made me cake) talking about her writing a piece on turning 60, something I think a man of her iconic status and social position would never have been asked to write. For all the cultural reasons we know about, women who turn 60 and don't look like we expect them to look at that age are a fascinating anomaly, but it's the 'for her age' tagline that is so dispiriting. Let's pretend that phrase has been banned by our new leader, Prime Minister Dolly Parton!

Nigella agreed to write the piece and be shot for the cover of the magazine for her birthday in January 2020. The feature was insightful, reassuring and soothing. If you are looking for a positive manifesto on ageing, I urge you to read it. Nigella's mother had died at 48, one of her sisters at 32 and her husband, John, at 47. Ageing was, she said, something we should give thanks for. We couldn't waste energy worrying about it; in fact, we should perhaps just ignore it. Life was easier as an older woman, she said, which I agree with – so much less looking around at others and people-pleasing. There was a freedom from judgement and a liberation to be enjoyed, which would be enhanced by nourishing our connections to others.

As a younger woman, Nigella wrote, she'd been like a fridge: the light only went on when someone else opened the door. Now, she said, she kept the light on all the time. That's something we can all look forward to.

101 Things That Will Make You Murderously Furious

~ **Parking apps** that don't work because you don't have a mobile signal while your teenagers are standing next to you yelling, 'Hurry up, Morag*, we don't have all day.' (*Insert parental nickname.)

~ **Lost iPhones:** Not yours, but your teenagers' phones and your elderly parents' phones. Dad, you didn't get mysteriously and silently mugged in the cheese aisle at Lidl, you just left your phone there.

~ **Hangovers** worse than anything Kingsley Amis could describe, and he once wrote about a hangover that left him 'spewed up like a broken spider-crab on the tarry shingle of the morning'. You feel worse than that. After one glass of wine. It is infuriating.

~ **Everyone on the Nextdoor app**, especially the ramblings of the Guinea Pig Alliance. More high-maintenance than cats, apparently. You have to put your phone down before you send angry missives about people's pets, which is unlike you.

~ **Millennials asking if you need to take a break in meetings.** You want to remind them that you once conducted a two-hour in-person meeting after 24 hours awake (that day you walked to work following a night at Heaven nightclub). So, no, you don't want a break, but you might like the meeting to end before *Escape to the Country* starts on telly.

~ **When your young daughter says, 'Where is Dad's claw hammer?'** Why is it Dad's? Why do tools only have masculine owners when you went to all that bother of not saying that for the whole of her childhood? You are almost constantly raging about the patriarchy waving 'your' wooden spoon around your kitchen.

~ **School WhatsApps** where they don't read the answers to questions and ask them multiple times, or you ask a question about World Book Day and someone answers asking for money for the end-of-term collection.

~ **Waiting for prescriptions:** The midlife prescription wait is endless: yours, your parents', your teens', your pets'.

~ **Hospital trips to be probed:** There seems to be a significant increase in medical probing after 50!

12

Big Time Sensuality

When a female dragonfly doesn't want to have sex she goes to extreme lengths: she fakes her own death. The she-dragon crashes to the floor and pretends to be dead to ward off any unwelcome erotic overtures after she has already mated, then she waits for Mr Dragon to fall asleep or go to work – I mean, fly away.

This idea of faking one's own death to avoid intimacy is not alien to women in midlife, I think. I don't know about you, but for me it felt like a fantasy option in the fluctuating chaos of perimenopause and menopause before the unfolding of our brighter second acts, before the awakening after the pause.

And maybe the idea of it sounds especially attractive to many women over 40 in long-term relationships that have morphed into the tense friendship of flatmates who bicker about whose turn it is to unload the dishwasher and which one of you gets to sit in their favourite spot on the sofa.

The subject of sex, libido and relationships in midlife is the one we return to most often on our podcast; it's the one our listeners say they find most complicated to navigate, as it is loaded with complex feelings and possibly years of cultural pressure. Solving our sex and love dilemmas is like wrestling with a physical and mental Rubik's Cube.

Hormones have a huge impact on the physical side of a woman's sex life. The decline in them can make intercourse painful, particularly for anyone who has suffered from vaginal atrophy (see page 241), which affects around 80 per cent of all women in midlife to some degree and will almost certainly make them wish to avoid sex (and the resulting urinary tract infections).

Sex is also culturally complex for midlife women in the UK because most of us a) were brought up by a spectacularly repressed generation of parents, and b) are perhaps weighed down by having nurtured our sexual identity throughout the confusing years of the ladette, *Bridget Jones's Diary*, *More!* magazine's Position of the Month, explicit newspaper agony aunts, lurid *News of the World* headlines and Nancy Friday's sexually fierce manual of female fantasies *My Secret Garden*. Ours was also the era when one-night stands were often defined as a 'good thing', or at least not unusual, and maybe even a goal to prove that our sexual appetites matched those of men, who were mistakenly thought to have bigger appetites in this area.

All these conflicting messages about sexual liberation often made me feel like sex had become a numbers game. There was so much information on it, especially as pornography was becoming so freely available. We assumed we should all be having sex all the time with all the people we could, to rack up our scores as younger women. I mean, how sexually unful-filled must we be if we hadn't tried a threesome or at least kissed someone of the same sex? And if we weren't engaging with multiple partners then we should at least be having sex morning, noon and night with the one partner we may have met after we left further education.

It was then assumed that when we got to our mid-forties Gen-X women probably stop having so much Samantha from *Sex and the City* sex because women having sex after that age – especially in their fifties or sixties – disappeared from our cultural references. Older women were deemed sexless unless they looked like Susan Sarandon, Julianne Moore or Helena Christensen in underwear adverts. And if you were not into men you had to be a 'lipstick lesbian' – a ridiculous phrase that seemed to pop up again and again over the years, which meant you had to look like Madonna kissing Britney Spears at the 2003 VMAs. It was all so baffling, running as it did alongside all the terrible and demeaning instructions for how to be bikini-body ready.

I say all this as a former editor of *Cosmopolitan* (who commissioned a story about a couple who had sex in space) and as a journalist specialising in 'women's interest stories'. I have therefore written more sex features than most, and I've talked to all manner of experts on this subject since the age of 19.

Once, when I was working for a tabloid newspaper, I was sent to interview a man who was taking his wife to court for forcing him into unwanted sexual intercourse. The headline the male editor wanted was 'Sex-mad wife' – because apparently this was such a surprising thing.

In the late '80s, if you were a single woman, it was aspirational to be a sex-mad glamour-model type, but, illogically, not normal to be sex mad if you were married. I pretended the couple had said no and returned to my desk wondering why sex was so fascinating to the British public, and particularly men. But even then, aged 23, I knew that if the wife had been over 40 I would not have been sent to ask for an interview: a sex-mad wife in her forties was an anomaly and a downer for circulation. No one wanted to think about that.

In comedian Amy Schumer's famous 2015 sketch 'Last F**kable Day', Julia Louis-Dreyfus, Tina Fey and Patricia Arquette act out a fake celebration of an actress being 'unfuck-able' on screen after she had hit her mid-fifties. Google it if you haven't seen it because it smartly and with great wit sums up the place we are in: how, deemed sexless after 50, we're finally allowed to guzzle ice cream in any quantity because our naked bodies don't need to hold any erotic charge anymore. It brilliantly skewers how the money men who greenlight most films and TV have long viewed and still view sex: as if it is just about what women look like.

Generation X in particular were very much sold the idea that youth, slimness and good sex were inextricably linked. The subliminal narrative around women seemed to be either a man-pleasing one (i.e. women who were always up for it in the same way as men were but only to please their men) or that sex was something that was 'done to us'. Those women who were having sex because they loved it were seen as rampant. There was no grey area in between for us normals who liked sex and were happy to say so but didn't want to do it all the time with all the people in all the positions. Perhaps our neurology was addled by growing up around all that Benny Hill humour and those sexy-nurse outfits for Halloween and that's why we generally accepted these narra-tives. When you look at in retrospect, all of it is so disturbing and utterly toxic.

However, as the former queen of Orgasm HQ (i.e. *Cosmo*), I can tell you now there is a sexual revolution on the way for women as they age. Rebellious Gen X has hit midlife, we're at a sexual checkpoint, we're erotically restless and we are vocal about it. Sex is on our to-do list, and it is about to be loaded into the emotional washing machine of midlife along with all the other stuff we're encountering.

There is a liberation for us in sex and sexuality – the rise of sex-toy sales for women tells you this, among other things. And I hear it ALL THE TIME, particularly from women over 40 who are having a lot of sex with men under 40. Younger men, it seems, are becoming the playground for our midlife desires.

I am bombarded (and I don't use that word lightly) with stories of women in their fifties and sixties who are sleeping with men three decades their junior on a regular basis (I have interviewed them – they are not anomalies, and they are very good in bed because confidence is an erotic superpower). Some previously heterosexual women are sleeping with other women, others are having affairs not because they are unhappy in their marriages but because they want more or better sex. Midlife women are paying to sleep with male and female sex workers, going to sex parties alone, enjoying orgies and taking their husbands to talk to sex therapists (to 'keep the flame alive', as we'd have headlined it at *Cosmo*). They are discovering masturbation daily using the new sugar-free lubes that don't cause diabolical thrush, they're taking testosterone and firing up their libidos once again, and those on HRT have become reacquainted with the sex lives they thought they'd lost.

Maybe some of us have at last realised that 'youthfulness' is not something younger women own. Maybe we are finally freeing ourselves from years of conditioning around our bodies and our sexual identity, and acknowledging that sex is about pleasure and not tied to what we look like? Maybe some women are happy that men desiring them for how they look is no longer on their list of wants – freedom from that can be joyous.

For many, this period of transition is a sexual melting pot, a time of self-definition. And single or newly single women have told me that releasing themselves from this Gen-X need to 'find the one' allows for more creativity and playfulness when it comes to sex, sexuality, love and relationships.

We have been told that being menopausal somehow signifies the end of our desirability (it is, after all, the least sexy of words). But it doesn't. That's only true if you see youth as the only sign of desirability, and we know it is not. It's far from over for us on the desire front.

Midlife is a dangerous age on this new sexual frontline – one when women can invite huge disruptions. We hear of many in our podcast community who start to explore all sorts of new ways of being, which may cause chaos in their personal lives.

In fact, I think society should perhaps be a little scared about the rising sexual power of midlife women today (especially as so many hundreds of women's libidos are being super-fuelled by HRT). A generation is getting its lust mojo on, and a ruckus will follow in other areas of our lives as result, I suspect, because good sex fuels good confidence too. Sexual confidence has powered parts of the patriarchy for centuries, and I think it is the missing part of the jigsaw for women. I, for one, am going to enjoy watching this sexual revolution unfold.

And of course we feel time is upon us – there are no second chances after midlife. This is your era of no periods, no babies, no sleepless nights with toddlers, no pregnancy risk, and it may open up an exciting new landscape to conquer. I think we're in the foothills of discovering this. Some of us haven't even opened the gate to the foothills, I know, but the key is in our pockets.

I can sense the change is coming. The increased sales in sex toys and the rise of sexually transmitted infections in the over-45s point to both liberating and potentially reckless new frontiers as people take risks when fertility is not a worry anymore. This is a time for your new sexual identity to be formed.

To find out more, I talked to sex coach Ruth Ramsay, because while all the evidence points to sexual adventures for midlife women I was also hearing sad stories about women who felt they would never get the sexual freedom they wanted, women who were stuck in erotic ruts and women who felt overwhelmed by the lack of sex in what otherwise seemed to be happy marriages. These women want more. Many others are super-charged by this new lust life they feel. Confusion reigns and of course everyone's experience is different, but this sexual charge in the air is now affecting us all in different ways, and I think there is an opportunity here to get something delicious back into our world and to harness our new sexual identities effectively.

Ruth, who is a former stripper, coaches 'singles, couples and thruples', as she puts it online. I trust her empathetic and realistic view of our sex lives at this age. She knows her stuff and she is in the eye of the storm age-wise.

'Men and women need to understand how limiting the templates we were given about sex are on our potential pleasure in all kinds of relationships, heterosexual or otherwise,' she tells me. 'For so long it hasn't been [about] our sexual desire, it has been about conforming to please the other person.

'Everyone needs to be better educated on their own anatomy and to really know what turns them on. We must try to abandon the idea [that] pleasure is linked to what we look like, because that isn't relevant; it is what our body feels like that is important.'

Ruth explains that culturally we are at a real disadvantage here. 'We are so uncomfortable in the UK when it comes to talking about sex,' she says. 'There is a mismatch for men and women around desire: women tell me they are broken in some way because they don't experience spontaneous desire, an ideal they have been sold in films and books. But that is normal.

'Research has shown 75 per cent of men (mostly younger men, though) may experience spontaneous desire, but most women almost never experience it. Doctors agree it is clinically normal for a woman never to feel spontaneous sexual desire.

What women need is a scenario to respond to; their desire is responsive depending on their environment, which is why I ask clients to plan their sexual activity; that is what the female brain needs.

'And I have found that as men age they are less spontaneous too, so they benefit from scheduling sexual activity, but before all that we have to find out what we enjoy, we have to find that nook inside ourselves that prompts our desire.'

When we asked our over-40 listeners about their sex lives in our private Facebook survey, 57 per cent said they owned a sex toy, 41 per cent wanted more sex, 39 per cent had it at least once a week and 75 per cent told us that intimacy and connection were the most important part of their sex lives, their biggest need. They were almost all masturbating, FYI.

So sex is critical for Gen X, and not just because we know orgasms are good for blood flow, which helps your hair grow among other things, but also because (and I can't repeat this enough) the quality of our relationships is the single most important predictor of a longer, healthier, happier life. Connection is key for all of us and when we lose this the ripple effect is huge. Loneliness is a killer. Sexual connection counts, especially with your partner. Touch is nourishing.

As your sexual identity changes, or possibly emerges, in midlife, it is due a playful upgrade, as one sex therapist we interviewed described it. And this is much-needed for many of the women I've spoken to on the show and for this book – those who have hit a sexual wall. There are a lot of couples who no longer have sex at all; indeed, the whispered 'it's been years' phrase is common among midlife WhatsApp threads. I know couples who have had five years of no sex in a long-term marriage or relationship. Some women may feel this is OK for them; they may take the Germaine Greer stance on it and feel relieved of the pressure to be or do something sexual. And it's

199

fine if that's you, but if a little niggle is there around the loss of your sex life then it could be beneficial to explore that further, and to take positive action.

So much is at play in the secret sex lives of couples. At this age and stage, women are often so overwhelmed with everything else going on in their daily domestic life that it's hard to go from cold to hot at the flick of a switch. If your day is caring for elderly parents, sorting school packed lunches and organising the laundry rotas so the PE kits are ready on time, you're not necessarily to going to be in the mood instantaneously.

This can cause discrepancies within relationships, as it is less hard for men to do this; according to sexual health experts I have interviewed, this transition from cold to hot is often easier for them to achieve, although many men do experience a slowing of their libido in midlife too.

The fact is that sex is dark and messy, full of contradictions. The loss of connection through sex is sad for many women, especially those who are physically in need of that release and those whose sexuality comes alive at this age. And what a life force sexuality is, however you choose to express it. In her 1978 essay 'Uses of the Erotic: The Erotic as Power', American writer and activist Audre Lorde called female sexuality 'the chaos of our strongest feelings'. Which is how it felt for me (after the right HRT prescription) – a new lease on life.

But perhaps releasing and exploring those sexual feelings is something else to be fearful of in midlife when there is already so much change happening that we must adapt to. I also wonder if we may feel 'greedy' for wanting more pleasure for ourselves instead of wanting to please our partners, which is probably part of our programming. These are difficult emotions to deal with, for sure.

This conundrum of no sex in long-lasting relationships was explored most thoroughly by psychotherapist Esther Perel in

her 2006 book *Mating in Captivity*, and if you watch her TED
Talk on the subject you get a sense of what a tricky thing it is
for long-term couples to maintain a happy sex life. She points
out that this need for security, stability and routine, which
satisfy us when we set up family life and create domestic intimacy, is often at odds with our need for desire or physical
intimacy; it is at odds with our erotic selves.

It's hard to be a best friend *and* a passionate lover, she says,
and adds that our imagination is the key to maintaining desire.
It's what marks us out from animals, who mate for procreation,
not pleasure.

'Toys and lingerie won't save you,' she says to the TED Talk
crowd, before explaining that our crisis of desire is a crisis of
imagination. Shifting our perception of the person who goes
through the recycling and berates us if we put a crisp packet
in there into a passionate partner is not easy. She advises that
couples cultivate some sexual privacy, that they have some
separation from each other. And that they ask themselves when
they find their partner most attractive. She explains that it will
usually be when they see them doing something they are
passionate about, or something separate from them.

As Ruth Ramsay puts it to me: 'The erotic equation is
attraction plus obstacle equals excitement. You need to add
an "obstacle" into your sex life. In my work with couples, I
may advise that perhaps the woman experiments with a sex
toy but tells her partner the time and place at home she may
be doing this behind a locked door where he cannot enter.
This obstacle and discussion around sex creates erotic charge.
Creating these obstacles can become a game. This relies on
you both being able to communicate about sex, though. We
start with that.'

It may seem counterintuitive but, according to Ruth, scheduling in time for sex can be transformative. 'A weekly diarised

sexual playtime is the most helpful thing a couple can do to reignite their sexual spark,' she says. 'I say to those I work with, "Just try it and if it hasn't helped within a month then come back to me." No one has ever come back to me.'

She also advises listening to podcasts about sex or sexual confessions for women. Beginning to bring the word into your life often liberates the mind. The brain is our biggest sex organ, but it needs to be exercised like a muscle.

Ruth also asks couples to identify their 'brakes and accelerators'. In other words, what really turns you off and on? A turn-off, or 'brake', might be the fact that your partner isn't supporting you in other areas of your life – after all, few of us want to have sex with a person they feel doesn't respect them or care about them. Talk about that (in a non-blaming way) and also then find out for yourself, on your own, what accelerates your sexual desire. Explore your own mind and body.

As Ruth says: 'I don't mean five minutes before sleep with your Womanizer sex toy! I mean really take time out for an evening alone with your body, the whole bath, relaxation, massage journey. Prepare yourself for sex; create a situation leading to desire.'

'Know yourself first' is what all sexual-health experts recommend, in my experience. Invest in the pleasure sex brings you as a woman (not a couple). When we interviewed Suzi Godson, the *Times*' sex columnist who has written many books on sex and sexuality for all ages, she told us sex was a form of communication for couples. That even though your libido fluctuates, a good sex life isn't always related to libido alone; it's more related to you and your general wellbeing, mentally and physically. We asked her for advice for couples struggling to stay sexually connected and she said it begins with fostering a more open dialogue between you.

'Sex is the first thing to go when relationships break down,' she said. 'Deciding to bring it back as a couple is a hugely positive step-change in a relationship. It's a choreographed dance between couples about needs, and the longer you leave it, the harder it is to revive a sex life.'

Suzi stressed, however, that there is always hope. 'If you start to focus on each other, sex can come back. This is a stage of life where women think of themselves in a more autonomous way, not as mothers, employees or wives. We begin to question our decisions and decide who we want to be. We may ask: "Am I out or am I back in?" and I would say if a woman decides she is in, there is a possibility of the sex becoming incredible, the connection being restored.'

As with so many intimacy issues, getting the words out in the first place is usually the hardest step. 'We don't really know how to talk about sex,' Suzi explained. 'Especially the men of this generation. My husband and I had counselling after we hit some problems and after talking about the other stuff, our sex life went through the roof. Deciding to be with each other in every sense of the word is sexually invigorating, but it can feel clumsy, weird and awkward at first to discuss the elephant in the room. If you don't, though, the elephant just gets bigger and bigger.'

When entrepreneur Anna Richards, who founded the erotic platform Frolicme in her early forties, came on *Postcards from Midlife* she told us that her midlife audience were women who'd opted for more adventure sexually – a growing number of midlifers who realised sex wasn't so much what your body looked like, but what it liked in terms of pleasure.

'Get to know yourself first is always my advice for those in long-term relationships who have lost the spark,' she told us. 'Buy that vibrator, experiment with understanding how your body responds to sexual pleasure. Connect with you.'

'Sex is emotional for women,' Ruth added. 'And it isn't ever over. You don't have to labour under the idea that if you haven't sorted your sex life out by your fifties it is over – it really isn't. Great sex is a possibility at all ages. Lengthen that view you may have of your sex life. It can be a forever thing.'

13

'What, This Old Thing? I've Had It for Years'

This chapter isn't for everyone. I am putting it here because it is a little cathartic and hopefully humorous. I am getting it off my chest (or off my 'Unmet Needs of Gen-X Women' WhatsApp thread), but you probably won't need to read this chapter unless you own one of these. I'm talking about husbands, of course! More specifically, much-loved, well-worn Generation-X husbands that you've had for aeons.

Many women around me find themselves on the Island of Midlife marooned with men we love (most of the time) who are of a similar age. Most of us have been with them since Tony Blair was prime minister. We know them inside out and here we are, in the messy middle bit weathering the stormy changes together. It's a unique collaboration, a comforting coupling.

I have been married for more than two decades, and we've been together for even longer than that. James and I met on a blind date at Oktoberfest, a beer festival, the oddest of events that neither of us would have gone to if a friend had not had spare tickets and been convinced we'd get along. We would never have been matched on Bumble. I doubt we would ever have met otherwise. I was woman's editor on a national newspaper and he was a management consultant working at a bank: we had nothing in common, but we did both love the film *Withnail and I* and, as it turned out, we only needed that one thing. It was an on–off affair at first and I had been clear about not really wanting to marry or have children. But our love affair whooshed along into a marriage that has robustly survived ever since that rainy Cornish day in October when we tied the knot.

I have never doubted that I married the right man. Obviously, I have wanted to kill him on numerous occasions (and vice versa, no doubt, though he is a mild-mannered fellow who is averse to confrontation). I knew he would be an amazing dad. I knew he would catch all of us if we fell. I was right.

Living with anyone – even the dog – for this length of time is a challenge, but living with the same human man continually is sometimes stressful, isn't it? Especially at the point in life when you may feel as if you're losing yourself or coming undone – 'the fuckening' as it was been referred to recently on social media, or the midlife place where we are occasionally 'very fuckstrated', as the TikTok meme goes.

Your patience decreases, your rage increases and your ability to tolerate imaginary ailments, loud sneezes, fast walking or long, complicated explanations about thermostats wanes. The hoarding of cardboard boxes and the keeping of broken electronic devices 'for the parts' are my particular bugbears.

But here you are, temporarily in an unexpected place, this weird town, with your other half who is probably going through his own midlife wobbles too. We will never hear the end of Mr Candy having to wear reading glasses, for example – a development he has taken extremely personally. Navigating all this is trickier than stacking the dishwasher, a job that both of you do wrong in the eyes of the other (knives pointed end down – how many times do I have to say this??).

There are, of course, better books than this one out there written by experts on relationships and the complications they may experience in midlife – I'll list some of them in the back for you (see page 236) and you can certainly listen to the experiences of the women on our podcast. Reading up on this subject could be extremely useful because, as mentioned in the previous chapter, I note that women often make cataclysmic decisions around their relationships in the chaos of the midpoint. The physical and psychological challenges we face in perimenopause and menopause are not a sensible or reliable backdrop for any major relationship changes. So, as I have said before, preparation is everything: if you know it is coming then perhaps you can seek help with managing your love life, or the love of your life, at this time, rather than being swept along in any kind of crisis that may occur. Perhaps you and your partner can talk about it together out loud, re-evaluating your habits and patterns of togetherness.

My husband was as lost as I was when my perimenopause symptoms hit in my late forties. Most Gen-X men are 'fixers' and he wanted a practical solution as the night terrors took hold and my mood plummeted out of the blue. He would look at me each day, subconsciously asking, 'Are you fixed yet?' feeling powerless. He tiptoed around me until I found out what was going on from Dr Louise Newson (see page 23), but it put a dent in our marriage because it is hard to live with a woman who is inexplicably losing her mind. The dynamic between us changed as I felt more vulnerable and illogically weaker. The only way through for us was to keep talking about it, and also to celebrate the bond we had in little ways every day – to be kinder to each other when the pressure mounted. Some of our rows were epic around this time, some were more muted and darker, and I can't help but feel it could all have been avoided if I had gone on HRT earlier, or at least understood why I felt the way I did. I was lucky my husband learned to listen to me properly as we discussed all these changes. I know many women aren't as supported, and that is heartbreaking.

And obviously men face their own midlife changes too; it might be a less physically dramatic experience than ours, but it can be just as painful, just as mentally messy. Many experts I've spoken to recommend a midlife relationship MoT, some talking therapy for couples to review where they are and what they may wish for next. Visions of the future are often very different in couples and that needs to be resolved or at least communicated. Everything is up in the air at this time, and it can be confusing for male partners as women navigate the newness of their changing identity post motherhood, post youth, post work, post losing their own mothers.

As a psychology expert once told me, 'Love is not a soft skill.' We think it will be easy, but it's hard. Maintaining love requires work. Love and loving people don't always come naturally; we are not necessarily taught how and it can be such an evolving learning curve. People change, family dynamics change, and throughout all that we must sustain close, loving relationships with energy and care. I have never taken this for granted and never will. My marriage is the best relationship of my life and now we are both in our mid-fifties the upkeep of it is even more important.

Time is running out. I may be increasingly intolerant of my husband's tendency to obsess about a recycling schedule. His constant humming may make me murderous, but when I wake up in the dead of night wondering which of us will die first I dig deep. Patience, positivity and gratitude: you're going to need all three in love and midlife.

Reader, I married him

In the meantime (and on a lighter note, for we need this too), it's time to brace yourself for a traditional, cliché-filled, old-school husband rant to make you laugh. So I hereby present you with the definitive list of things that annoy midlife wives about men they have been with for more seasons than *Friends* was on telly. If I was narrating it in the manner of David Attenborough, I would note that many of these habits occur after the human male has passed 50: late-onset humming is particularly common, it seems.

And before you write in to complain, I am of course aware that if I was a man writing this chapter about my middle-aged wife, I'd most certainly be 'cancelled', but until the pendulum swings nearer to equality (it's nudging towards the centre at an irritatingly glacial pace), I think it's OK for me to throw this out there. It's my turn to gently make fun of men using predictable gender generalisations; this is, after all, our 'lived experience', as the modern catchphrase goes. I don't offer this list to diminish the men/man in our lives, though they are a sensitive bunch; I have popped it here to acknowledge the lifelong patience needed when you spend so much time with one person.

This affectionate list, gifted to me by our wonderful podcast Facebook group, doesn't mean we love our husbands or partners less (I share an underwear drawer with mine, that's how close we are), and we are well aware that they could produce an equally impressive list of our annoying traits, and that there are always exceptions to the rule. You can skip it if you're refreshingly single, or 'newly liberated', as someone described it to me, but, if you are not, it is here to save you furiously typing these things into your phone in a supermarket car park for the benefit of your girlfriends. And it's here, as is everything in this book, to make you feel less alone. For a while I thought I was the only woman becoming ridiculously intolerant of minor things. Turns out I am not, and I found it endearing, the honesty of all these midlife women getting this stuff off their chest and going about their day feeling a little lighter, and hopefully a bit more tolerant of the men in their lives, as a result.

101 Things That Could Get Midlife Husbands Killed by the Women Who Love Them Most

~ 'The thing he does with his fingers (drumming them together at the top) that reminds me of *The Simpsons'* Mr Burns.'

~ 'Dad noises: habitual throat clearing, groans, grunts accompanying physical exertion. Particularly when getting up.'

~ Asking me why our cats and dog are doing things, or what they want, as if I have a telepathic connection to them.'

~ 'Being unable to close a door quietly. Why must they all be slammed?'

~ 'He has about five things wrong with him every night and morning, and frequently asks me what could be wrong with him. I have no medical training.'

~ 'Walking so fast we can't keep up: he used to do it when the kids were small on their way to school, and I once saw him halfway up the road and the three of them trailing behind chasing him to school.'

~ 'Watching Facebook reels on his tablet out loud while I'm trying to watch TV. I've taken to turning the TV off till he realises.'

~ 'Cutting a fresh block of cheese and it looking like he's had a fight with it, even though he's a civil engineer, then putting it back in the fridge unwrapped where it can air-dry in peace.'

~ 'Explaining things as if I'm a halfwit. Usually incorporating the phrase, "If you understand what I'm saying . . ."'

~ 'We can't drive past a petrol station without my husband reading out the price of diesel and comparing it to the last five we drove past over the last five days!!!'

~ 'Insisting on telling me his regime for the central-heating-system temperatures, and timings thereof.'

14

Tuck 'n' Roll

One of my favourite women is a no-nonsense, tall, glamorous blonde just a few years older than me. Let's call her Joyce. She was once my boss. When we first started to work together people were taking bets on how long our relationship would last, assuming two strong female personalities would never get on and that one of us would have to triumph over the other – the usual narrative for two forthright women working along-side each other.

I knew within minutes of meeting Joyce that we would be friends for the rest of our lives. Her unbreakable spirit and her ability to see an upside in everything was incredibly alluring to me. I had not met anyone like her. She was a unique female, one of the best. Fiercely loyal, non-judgemental, relentlessly honest, a problem solver of the highest order. She really knew who she was; her identity was solid, unquestioned in her own mind, and this felt like the holy grail to me, part of the secret to strong womanhood. Meeting her in my mid-forties was like finding a rope to hold onto in a twister.

I particularly loved Joyce's stories of growing up in Nova Scotia, one of which has given me a lesson pertinent to midlife that is worth sharing.

When Joyce's dad drove her to school in his unpredictable old car he'd have to keep the car moving and the engine running as he dropped her at the gates. He couldn't stop or the cranky vehicle would not start again. In the freezing-cold winters this became an easier task for the family because of the large snow drifts gathered on the road outside the school. Joyce's dad would slow down, heading towards a drift, and ask young Joyce to open the car door and hurl herself out of the moving vehicle into the snow. As she did so he would yell, 'Tuck 'n' roll, Joyce, tuck 'n' roll!' She'd land softly in the white stuff, pause for a moment, then get up and shake herself off before heading into school for the day. You, my friends, are at the tuck-'n'-roll stage of life. You have to tuck 'n' roll before landing in that drift, pausing (as we have discussed, the pause is important – see Chapter 6) and then dusting yourself off to head into stage two of this wonderful life you are leading, or will lead.

The losses may have been numerous in this midlife quest to form, find or consolidate your identity, but if you enter the next stage prepared, perhaps it will be easier. I wish I had known everything about perimenopause and menopause before they had happened – I wish I'd known what would happen to my mind and body, how I would feel as a woman as I aged. It would have saved time. I would have felt less alone, less like there was something wrong with me, if I had known this was all perfectly normal. I would have known what to do. There would have been less grumbling and less fury or resistance. I would have tuck 'n' rolled with the shape-shifting of my identity.

That is why I wrote this book. It is full of things I believe all midlife women need to know. Hopefully you've learned much from the previous chapters, taken in some ideas that could help you grasp the positivity of this new situation you find yourself in. Because there is plenty of positivity to be found.

When I interviewed the Booker Prize-winning writer Margaret Atwood in London in 2019 I asked her if she enjoyed getting older. She was 80 at the time. She said: 'I have enjoyed everything. Why not?'

A sage piece of advice, indeed: enjoy everything. Why not?

The middle bit really is juicy for finding out who you want to be. It is a time for rebellious hope, a time for optimism, a time for magnificence. Midlife is ripe with giddy possibilities – a release, a spirited liberation, a new energy, a flourishing new you, or just some peace (that came to me in my mid-fifties, but you can get it earlier if you are prepared, which hopefully you are now).

Optimism becomes a verb at this point, because, as Julia Samuels says, 'hope is the alchemy of change'. This is not a crisis, though it may feel like it occasionally; this is an opportunity – an opportunity arising out of ongoing change and transformation. You are not lacking anything, you are gaining things. You have had many identities and shaped some of them to make others comfortable with them. You don't have to do that anymore. You can be the real you. Maybe you are not falling apart as you thought you were; perhaps you're unravelling to straighten yourself out and now you're coming back together stronger.

You can choose who you are now that you understand that change is and always will be constant and you have no control over that. I think you'll find an even happier you by accepting who you are, being less reactive and less judgemental, and more curious, more open.

I certainly have. I have felt a huge sense of letting go as I have moved through this void of confusion between older and younger, this transformation and personal evolution. What comes next will be as good as I make it. And if it's not, I can deal with that too.

I feel there is less leaning in, less bending around things that don't suit you, but also more acceptance of difficult situations and feelings. It is quite a relief not to have to be all things to all people, not to have it all anymore. It's a relief to relinquish any attachment to the status of previous roles you had, to be softer, more vulnerable. To explore more, and to fail when you need to and to see the grey areas when before you would have seen black and white. I don't need to 'get a grip' of anything anymore.

I feel more awake to each day, more observant now that I have slowed down and embraced being less manic. I am more creative and playful. I can feel this melancholia drifting away, or at least slipping out of sight, now that I know what is going on. There's no more creeping sadness, just a slow, creeping gladness. I am burning with new insight. I can see the tran-quillity on the horizon. I can sit with the discomfort of change. I can usually observe (and ignore) the shitty committee in my head. I can feel the sadness of impending endings without them bleeding into the sunrise of a new day. I have an idea of who I want to be today (and it may change tomorrow – nothing is set in stone now). I've discovered that the spaces in between things happening are just as important as, if not more than, what happens next. And I am, of course, grateful just to be here.

Good luck to you

They say the darkest hour is the one before the dawn; midlife feels a little like a new dawn to me. It may drop you into your darkest hour yet, but, like an animal coming out of hibernation, you'll soon turn your face to the sun and thaw, softening with relief and liberation in her optimistic warmth. You won't feel lost or alone anymore. You'll have the hope of a new era coming. And perhaps you will realise that you are all the women you have ever been. They echo through you, forming the woman you are today and the woman you will evolve into tomorrow. Those women are there for you, like all of us, so you are never alone. It really is all going to be OK. And if it's not OK, you'll be OK with that. I promise, because . . .

You're Princess Leia blasting a hole in that vent yelling, 'Somebody has to save our skins!' You're Alanis Morissette singing that everything is just fine, fine, fine in 'Hand in My Pocket'. You're Sandra Bullock driving that bus in Speed. *You're Elizabeth*

Hurley in her Versace safety-pin dress. You're Naomi Campbell getting up after tumbling on the catwalk in 11-inch Vivienne Westwood heels. You're Julia Roberts telling the sales assistants they've made a 'big mistake' in Pretty Woman. *You're Madeleine Albright the day she was appointed the first ever female secretary of state. You're Erin Brockovich telling the court, 'I don't need pity, I need a pay check.' You're welder Jennifer Beals auditioning in* Flashdance. *You're Madonna in* Desperately Seeking Susan *drying her armpits in that New York restroom. You're Helen Mirren telling Michael Parkinson that women can be serious actors even if they have breasts. You are Ruth burning down her marital house in TV drama* The Lives and Loves of a She-devil. *You are Tina Turner singing 'Proud Mary' at Barcelona's Olympic Stadium. You are Sigourney Weaver as Ripley in every* Alien *film. You are Sarah Connor in* Terminator. *You're Diana Ross singing 'I'm Coming Out'. You're Flo-Jo winning three golds at the 1988 Olympics. You're Carmela Soprano teasing that hot priest. You are Buffy the Vampire Slayer and Monica from* Friends *rolled into one. You're Princess Diana on the red carpet in her skin-tight, off-the-shoulder Oscar de la Renta 'revenge dress' . . . and you are Shirlie Holliman and Dee C. Lee in their white bikinis walking towards the Club Tropicana pool, enjoying the fun and sunshine, because there's enough for everyone.*

101 Things Only Midlife Women Know: My 'Are You Having Fun Yet?' Playlist

'Pure Shores' – All Saints
'You Oughta Know'– Alanis Morissette
'Killing Me Softly with His Song' – Fugees
'Creep' – Radiohead
'Smells Like Teen Spirit' – Nirvana
'No Scrubs' – TLC
'Loaded' – Primal Scream
'Bittersweet Symphony' – The Verve
'Born Slippy' – Underworld
'Let's Talk About Sex' – Salt-N-Pepa
'Purple Rain' – Prince
'The Whole of the Moon' – The Waterboys
'Africa' – Toto
'Come On Eileen' – Dexys Midnight Runners
'Rio' – Duran Duran
'Once in a Lifetime' – Talking Heads
'Glory Box' – Portishead
'Big Time Sensuality' – Björk
'All I Wanna Do' – Sheryl Crowe
'Unfinished Symphony' – Massive Attack
'Wannabe' – Spice Girls
'Club Tropicana'/'Young Guns (Go for It)' – Wham! (all Wham! songs actually)
'Common People' – Pulp
'Parklife' – Blur
'Torn' – Natalie Imbruglia
'Constant Craving' – k.d. lang
'Piazza, New York Catcher' – Belle and Sebastian
'Novocaine for the Soul' – Eels

15

101 Things
Midlife Women Can Do

This is a list of ideas, some wisdom gathered from the women around me, from the women I have interviewed, the women I have observed from afar, the women I love, the women ahead of me in life (our elders) and the women who support us professionally and personally. I can't speak to the specifics of your circumstances – we have all been through different times, different joys, different dramas, different childhoods and backgrounds – but these general thoughts below may lead you towards an optimism that will make your second act, after the pause, easier and even more enjoyable.

It's not a to-do list, there is no test at the end of it, you can't 'do it wrong'. There is no recipe for living, as we know. Some of the below may not work for you and you may find a few bits of it unpalatably trite (you have been warned!), but all of it comes from the experience of experts and from women who have found that a more curious mindset has improved their midlife journey. Please remain open to these ideas if they are new to you – don't dismiss them out of hand with your Act One mindset, because you may not think like that anymore!

Embrace a softening: As you no longer need to bend around anyone or anything anymore, lean into a kinder way of treating yourself. Dump the Gen-X martyr mindset, the endurance mantra. You can't outrun your own vulnerability, so melt into the softness of it and show it. It's not a sign of weakness or a loss of strength, it's a blanket to keep you warm and protect you during what lies ahead.

Love/like/respect yourself more: I know! Don't groan. I mean it; how can anyone love you if you don't love you? To expect them to is presumptuous, illogical and probably won't happen. The task here, though, is to know yourself better. That's where the peace lies.

Remember, you can't outsmart or avoid uncertainty, and midlife is peak uncertainty. There is no controlling it with rigidity. There is no avoiding it either, no putting-your-hands-over-your-ears or humming and numbing your way out of feeling it. If something messy, tricky, painful or grief-inducing is going to happen, the chances are it will happen now, so you'll have to face those feelings. Brené Brown's blog post 'The Midlife Unraveling' describes this perfectly and, even if you are teeth-sucking cynically at the mention of her name, it is worth reading. Getting to really know yourself through this uncertainty is the hardest part of our midlife conundrum: Brown likens the middle bit of life to a nasty street fight with the universe. This description very much resonated with me.

Write it down: May God forgive me but journaling is 'a thing' and it may help. Do jot your feelings down because it is better out than in, and, if you don't, you can't join the dots and see a pattern in the stories you are telling yourself. And holding it all in is very bad. Can we just think of another word than journaling?

Curate your world: From the social media you read, to the people, to the news you absorb: ask, 'Is this serving me well? Or is the chatter too negative, reinforcing the things I tell myself on the dark days, backing up that shitty committee in my mind?' If it's the latter, step away from it. Change the routine and curate a more positive world around you. Feed yourself with the good stuff. Review it every morning.

Stop worrying about 'everyone': As in, 'everyone' needs me to do/be/say this. Everyone won't like me; everyone is happier if I . . . 'Everyone' can look after themselves. Their business is not your business anymore.

Find awe in the day: What gives you small bumps of joy? Is it nature, music, laughter? There is science behind the theory that experiencing 'awe' makes us feel happier, but also it is bloody obvious. Research has shown that music and gardening should be a social prescription for those battling illness. These are big 'awe' suppliers. What could yours be?

Seek out moments of alonement: This isn't about being lonely, more being at ease in your own, solitary company (see page 65). Learn to breathe properly in your alonement. Maybe this is a few moments standing outside each morning. This time will calm the parasympathetic nervous system (a network of nerves that relaxes the body), which is like strengthening a muscle. Learning to be alone is a good thing for overwhelmed midlife women. Take it slowly.

BUT . . . also find your tribe: Social interaction will keep you feeling alive, awake and happy. Find new friends and actively nourish the good ones you have got. One of the biggest predictors of a long life is social interaction. Award-winning *New York Times* author Dan Buettner studied the five places in the world where people live the longest and healthiest lives, so-called Blue Zones. He came to five conclusions for longer life: we should eat less processed food, move regularly throughout the day (not high-impact malarkey; he was very definite about that NOT being good for us), get proper sleep, cultivate a strong sense of purpose and, crucially, find a circle of four to five friends you can depend on. So work out who is in your friendship front row. Women who had coped with cancer told me that a diagnosis often sorted the line-up easily, so imagine who would be there for you, whose company you can't live without, who makes you laugh. Do it as a matter of some urgency. And find some new friends too. I found my new tribe swimming outside, I found some on Instagram, I said yes to meeting strangers for a coffee. I made an effort, and it works. I followed up messages with phone calls. I was present for my new friends and nourishing for my old friends (I hope).

Step forward into growth, not backwards into the safety of old routines. It feels uncomfortable because it is, but to feel less lost you need to go through this emotional transitional pain. This means perhaps not accepting roles too similar to the ones you stepped out of; instead, opt for some 'nothing', then something else perhaps. Don't step into the same type of relationships, the same jobs, the same situations. Don't repeat the same parenting patterns that didn't serve you well. Self-check on this constantly.

Remember all those women you have been before? They were great, really they were. You may feel like you can't mention them now because you are perhaps a shadow of them in midlife, but you should overcome that. Celebrate the previous you a bit more. Relive her successes in your mind. Talk about her out loud. We often look back and see the ways we failed, rather than celebrating the times we did something well. Midlife is a time for reliving the highs of your past, which will be useful to your future. Make a list.

Learn when your energy times are. I am hopeless between 2 and 5 p.m. – this is my least effective part of the day, so I plan around it. I know not everyone can, but if you can then do. The hours between 6 and 8 a.m. are my most effective. I do my best everything then. I am all about the sunrises now; each one feels like a mini-adventure – I see several of them each week. This is probably what Oprah meant when she told me (in person!) to 'find your frequency': you're a different machine from everyone else, so adapt the day to suit you best where you can.

Attend to your past: Re-examining past events and your response to them helps provoke an awakening. I have watched immensely strong women who've been through quite shocking experiences, or who've spent a lifetime caring for others, coping with unmentionable situations and forgetting to acknowledge what they have lived through when they hit midlife. Don't forget to honour your previous experiences.

Feelings are not facts: Beware of the stories you tell yourself. Don't conflate feeling with fact. Feeing something – say, powerlessness – doesn't mean it is so. Stop to read that again and think about it. Don't turn against yourself in this way. The language you use around yourself is important, so resist the urge to criticise yourself out loud. Get out of the habit of doing that. Remove the negativity. And remember, what you are feeling may not be factually what is happening, so keep examining that.

Your appearance is probably the least interesting thing about you, so don't overthink it or worry about it to your detriment. It's a time thief and right now you need all the time you can get.

Embrace not knowing: Step into the pause between young and old, the fertile void I have written about (see Chapter 6). Leap into that liminal space with an open, curious mind. Abandon 'should', abandon previous routines in this plotless midpoint. Feel all the feelings here. Process the grief of the living losses around you. Be grateful that you have the time to age. Many don't get the chance.

Take up yoga and give it time to work. I hate myself for writing this, but it is true. Just do it. Call it 'my stretches' if the very word 'yoga' still feels too elite, too smug, too middle-class for you.

Look after your gut: That microbiome is like a garden that needs tending. Nurture it well and everything will be easier. We interviewed the charismatic gut-health guru Professor Tim Spector on the podcast and I read much of his research on how the gut is viewed scientifically as the second brain. It controls inflammation and inflammation is bad; it triggers all kinds of ailments and he advises eating 30 different types of plant a week (this includes herbs and, joyously, coffee). I felt much more energetic when I adopted this advice.

Cold showers: A game changer for me. Start slow, with maybe 15 to 30 seconds, and then build up. Gradually you will feel as if you are being given a *Pulp Fiction*-like shot of adrenaline each morning. It's not for everyone, but it's worth a try to kick-start your feel-good times. Ditto cold-water swimming.

Develop coping strategies for when you feel overwhelmed. What can you do when you feel out of sorts, mojo-less or as if you are being dragged into a darker place? It could be small amounts of exercise each day, a 10-second breathing routine, gathering with close friends, eating well, sleeping well, time with the dog, nature. Find what works for you by experimenting, so these strategies gradually become habits or rituals to guide you through the trickier times, of which there will be a few. It shouldn't be booze, cake or chocolate, but it could be dancing. Or maybe just shake it off, like dogs do after a stressful moment – a quick shake works wonders, I find. Discover what the experts call 'regulating behaviours' – activities to help you cope with difficult emotions. Reading works as well. Write them down as a list so you remember to do one each time you need to. And then make them non-negotiable parts of your daily or weekly routine. They will be grounding moments for you.

Nap: There is something to be said for the power of a good nap. Many women spoke to us about this on the podcast. It doesn't work for me, but it may for you. Try a 20-minute snooze during the day or a lie-down. Don't get under the covers, though – that way lunacy lies.

Quit moaning: Often our endurance mindset makes us find examples of things to endure that we don't have to endure; it is an unfortunate habit. Only one person is responsible for your happiness at this point, and it is you. Don't go for the grumble on the WhatsApp, don't shout at the telly, just keep out of negative threads. Keep it positive or don't say anything at all.

Think small: Small changes, small steps, small things to add in. Don't be tempted to think about huge change or achievements, or exhausting reinventions, as a way to stop you unravelling; they may be distractions from the feelings. Start by adding small routine changes to your day. It's the same with proactive change: do one small thing, then another. Otherwise, it is all too overwhelming. Take 'mouse steps', as someone once advised me.

Review your routines: Move the furniture regularly, change the colours, look for visual joy in your home. Clear out old things that are broken or remind you of other times you'd rather forget. Stuff can't go with you when you die – although I am concerned my husband may chuck all the phone chargers and mascaras I have hidden to stop my teens using them into the coffin when I go! Only keep what you use or love. Only keep what brings you joy. It's less stuff than you would think.

Money, money, money: Make it your business. Many women reach this stage of life and have no idea how to handle it, then they feel ashamed and don't have the confidence to sort out issues. I interviewed several financial advisors who told me their female midlife clients had handed running the money over to male partners, believing men were better at it, without any evidence for this being factually accurate. Women have up to 40 per cent less money at retirement on average than men,[11] so it doesn't look as rosy for us in midlife. You MUST make a date in your diary for a money MoT (especially if you are in the process of a divorce). Most financial advisors will save you the cost of a consultation – or financial diagnosis session, as they call it – with the advice they give. You should be reviewing your pension strategy, ensuring you generally have three to six months' worth of money in your current account (any more than that should be invested) and planning for a specific future rather than general goals. This means budgeting for uni fees, for downsizing, for looking after elderly parents. It's the time of life to get a financial grip. And there are debt-advice charities that can help you for free if you are in dire straits. There is a way through the money maze, but you have to purposefully find it.

Mindfully make new happy family memories: Do this on purpose, consciously. If, for example, you have a tricky time with your teens and bad things were said and done on both sides, apologise well the next day when the heat has died down (how you apologise is far more important than the initial disagreement), and then carefully plan to make new memories with them. It is never too late to reconnect with anyone or anything. Ruptures are not the problem, it's how you repair them that is important. And with adolescents this can be done with simple day-to-day moments of connection as well as purposefully making new memories with them. This doesn't always have to mean grand gestures, according to the parenting experts I've interviewed. You want to aim for what they call 'pot-plant parenting' when it comes to teenagers, which is less stressful all round in midlife: just being obviously available to them in the room and being interested in them and actively listening to them, instead of offering your own experiences or solutions to their problems. And always talk side by side, never face to face. When you have got the hang of not being their problem solver, then you can plan some new family memories.

Tell yourself it will be OK: 'What a ridiculous thing to say,' you may sigh, but relief is a placebo for your plastic brain, which undergoes many neurological changes in midlife as hormones fluctuate and disappear. So train your brain by speaking the words and it might just subconsciously shift your thinking towards believing it will be OK. Saying it out loud regularly may trick you into a calmer, more positive mindset, which is ripe for problem solving.

Find out more about 'your essential self': My guess is she is not in a wine glass or a biscuit tin or a big job, in intense exercise or a new relationship or any kind of drama. She is whispering to you internally, so listen to her, as you would to a friend telling you how she feels. We often hide who we really are to fit into the world we live, mould ourselves around others as we fulfil all our roles, but the real you is still in there somewhere and midlife is the time to liberate her and bring her to life again. Trusting your intuition will help you do this. Who is the 'soul of you'?

Transformation, reinvention, regeneration is not the end destination, not a goal – that is too performative a way to look at it – it is an external metric. Transformation is learning to be at peace with everything so that new ideas can weave their way through the forest of all your thoughts and feelings. By this I mean enjoy the transformation bit even when it is painful; I don't mean write 'reinvention' on your to-do list. If it happens, it happens, but enjoy the journey and stop judging yourself along the way.

Hold on to the threads of older women's positive stories tightly – those who always see the upside, the non-moaners. They will pull you through.

Write a list of 100 things you love: By the time you get to 60 or so you'll be discovering what really excites and moves you (see page 171). Take time to do this gradually and start with small, everyday things.

Say no: Set those boundaries at work and at home with the quiet power of midlife thinking. Just say no. It may not be popular, but time is running out, so say no to the things you don't want to do. And that's the reason for saying no: because you don't want to do it. You don't always have to explain yourself. It's such a relief when you do this. I have some tricky relatives who always want meetings in their home, yet every time we do this it goes wrong, and I have finally learned to say no to that venue. If we meet, we meet in a café and the whole process is much easier. I set a boundary, which removed an enormous amount of stress from me at midlife.

Therapy: I think it is worth trying it if you can afford it, particularly for specific family issues or to stop yourself repeating patterns that may be making you unhappy. It is good on rupture and repair, good on ways to reconnect on your own terms, good on grief and letting go. And it's helpful in navigating our new roles in midlife. I have tried it twice and found it extremely useful. It takes the lid off the anger pot too. It's maintenance of the mind; you could think of it in the same way you consider an MoT for the car.

Language is important: Age is just a number, so don't collude with society when it lays down the law on what you are supposed to be at a certain age. Avoid saying things like 'having a senior moment' or laughing at jokes about the perimenopause 'sounding like a Nando's hot sauce'. Try not to fuel the fire of derision and disappointment. It's diminishing.

Say hello to tranquillity: She is your new emotion. Seek her out and practise sitting with her. It's all part of slowing down. And slowing down is good because it refuels you and gives you the energy for anything you want to use it for – the planning of your magnificent midlife adventure perhaps?

And talking of adventure, have a few: In the softening and slowing-down you will find the space to nurture a dream; the seeds of ideas you planted will grow in that space. Slowing down doesn't mean opting out of epic challenges that take you out of your comfort zone. When I was 48 I swam the length of Lake Geneva in an amateur relay team. It's 70km, so like swimming the Channel and then back again. Six of us swam it with a swim coach. I couldn't do front crawl before I accepted this challenge, which is regarded as one of the world's longest and most difficult swims. But it changed my life. It gave me courage and confidence to take into other areas, and it gave me memories I know will slip into my mind in future when hours of front crawl (often in the dark) probably won't be possible. I will always have Geneva: my midlife adventure. More will follow in this slower, more optimistic stage of life.

Magical thinking: Consider the woo-woo. I have spent a career avoiding star signs and raising eyebrows at psychics. I am the first person in the room to say, 'I'm going to stop you there . . .' if a stranger mentions my aura or feng shui, but . . . I have come to realise as I have matured that perhaps there are small pockets of joy to be found in the inexplicable bits of life, or in a positive pep talk at least. Maybe believing in something bigger than you opens your mind to accepting that you can't control it all. Maybe it makes you think differently. I highly recommend author Elizabeth Gilbert as your guide on magical thinking. And entrepreneur Mo Gawdat. Just sayin' . . .

Helpful List for Midlife Women

Here are a few recommendations and resources that I've found useful – podcasts, books, websites, etc. – to help you, inspire you, inform you further on the intricacies of this midlife minefield. (Sorry if I have left anyone out – as we know, my memory isn't what it used to be!)

Podcasts

~ *Postcards from Midlife*: Our podcast, hosted by me and Trish Halpin. They don't call us the 'Menopausal Morecambe and Wise' for nothing! We hope our wise, funny guests bring new thinking and new possibilities to your midlife journey. And that our experts arm you with the information needed to help you embrace this stage of life with optimism.
~ *The Dr Louise Newson Podcast*
~ *Menopause Whilst Black: The Podcast* by Karen Arthur (follow her on Instagram too)
~ *The Menopause and Cancer Podcast* with Dani Binnington

Online

~ Balance app from Newson Health Research and Education, with symptom tracker (free to download): balance-menopause.com

~ The Menopause Charity – for information and advice on the menopause: themenopausecharity.org

~ Professor Vikram Sinai Talaulikar – follow for women's health updates in midlife: Twitter @VikramSinai

~ The Tweakments Guide – Alice Hart-Davis's website for any advice on cosmetic surgery: thetweakmentsguide.com

~ Feel Good with Lavina – for sensible exercise routines with wellness coach Lavina Mehta MBE: feelgoodwithlavina.com

~ Michelle Griffith-Robinson OLY – former Olympian and life coach: michellegriffithrobinsonoly.co.uk; Instagram @michellegriffithrobinson

~ Liz Earle Wellbeing – particularly good for nutrition advice: lizearlewellbeing.com

~ Wellbeing of Women – women's health charity. Check out their amazing YouTube videos of women discussing their menopause: wellbeingofwomen.org.uk

~ Dr Nighat Arif – NHS GP specialising in women's health: TikTok @drnighatarif; Instagram @drnighatarif

~ Menopause Mandate – information-based campaign group lobbying government: menopausemandate.com

~ The Latte Lounge – advice and information for midlife women, including a podcast with Katie Taylor: lattelounge.co.uk

~ Hylda – wellness platform for midlife women: hyldalife.com

~ Diane Danzebrink – menopause expert and activist who runs #MakeMenopauseMatter: dianedanzebrink.com

~ Owning Your Menopause – menopause fitness with expert Kate Rowe-Ham: owningyourmenopause.com

~ Davina McCall – the OG menopause warrior for us all: thisisdivina.com; Instagram @davinamccall; Twitter @ThisisDavina; Facebook en-gb.facebook.com/Davina McCall

~ WalkActive – website for fitness in midlife by Joanna Hall: walk-active.com

~ Rachel Schofield – career coach: rachelschofield.co.uk

~ Women Returners – career advice: womenreturners.com

~ Miss Lolly – financial advisor Lisa Conway-Hughes: misslolly.com

~ Money Saving Expert – Martin Lewis: moneysavingexpert. com

~ Follow Carolyn Harris, MP to support the work of the All Party Parliamentary Group on Menopause: Twitter @carolynharris24; menopause-appg.co.uk

~ Jo Divine – sex toys and advice on sexual health: jodivine. com; Instagram @jo.divine

~ Dr Naomi Potter's regular Instagram Lives with Lisa Snowdon are fact-filled and helpful: Instagram @drmenopausecare

~ Brené Brown's story 'The Midlife Unraveling' is a must-read: https://brenebrown.com/articles/2018/05/24/the-midlife-unraveling

~ MegsMenopause – Menopause and women's health advice curated by Meg Mathews: megsmenopause.com

~ Esther Perel's interviews and masterclasses are helpful for relationships: estherperel.com

~ Gut expert Professor Tim Spector specialises in menopausal women: tim-spector.co.uk

~ Elaine Kingett – award-winning writer specialising in adventures as we age: elainekingett.co.uk

~ Judy Glickman Lauder's work: judyglickmanlauder.com

Books

~ *Big Magic: Creative Living Beyond Fear* by Elizabeth Gilbert (Bloomsbury, 2015)

~ *Every Family Has a Story: How We Inherit Love and Loss* by Julia Samuel (Penguin Life, 2022)

~ *Everything You Need to Know About the Menopause (But Were Too Afraid to Ask)* by Kate Muir (Gallery UK, 2022)

~ *Five Arguments All Couples (Need to) Have: And Why the Washing Up Matters* by Joanna Harrison (Souvenir Press, 2022)

~ *Food for Life: The New Science of Eating Well* by Tim Spector (Jonathan Cape, 2022)

~ *Hagitude: Reimagining the Second Half of Life* by Sharon Blackie (September Publishing, 2022)

~ *How to Heal a Broken Heart: From Rock Bottom to Reinvention* by Rosie Green (Orion Spring, 2021)

~ *How to Stay Sane* by Philippa Perry (Macmillan, 2012) (this book features genograms)

~ *Mating in Captivity: Reconciling the Erotic and the Domestic* by Esther Perel (HarperCollins, 2006)

~ *M-Boldened: Menopause Conversations We All Need to Have* edited by Caroline Harris (Flint, 2020)

~ *Menopausing: The Positive Roadmap to Your Second Spring* by Davina McCall with Dr Naomi Potter (HQ, 2022)

~ *Menopause: All You Need to Know in One Concise Manual* by Dr Louise Newson (J.H. Haynes & Co. Ltd, 2019)

~ *Menopocalypse: How I Learned to Thrive During Menopause and How You Can Too* by Amanda Thebe (Greystone Books, 2020) (good on health and fitness)

~ *Money Lessons: How to Manage Your Finances to Get the Life You Want* by Lisa Conway-Hughes (Penguin Life, 2019)

~ *Midlife Bites: Anyone Else Falling Apart, Or Is It Just Me?* by Jen Mann (Ballantine Books Inc., 2022)

~ *Out of Time: Midlife, If You Still Think You're Young* by Miranda Sawyer (HarperCollins, 2016)

~ *Perimenopause Power: Navigating Your Hormones on the Journey to Menopause* by Maisie Hill (Green Tree, 2021)

~ *Preparing for the Perimenopause and Menopause* by Dr Louise Newson (Penguin Life, 2021)

~ *Quilt on Fire: The Messy Magic of Midlife* by Christie Watson (Chatto & Windus, 2022)

~ *Skincare: The New Edit* by Caroline Hirons (HQ, 2021) (helps with a midlife skin reboot)

~ *Spoon Fed: Why Almost Everything We've Been Told About Food Is Wrong* by Tim Spector (Vintage, 2022)

~ *STILL HOT!: 42 Brilliantly Honest Menopause Stories* by Kaye Adams and Vicky Allan (Black & White Publishing, 2020)

~ *The Bridge: A Nine-step Crossing into Authentic and Wholehearted Living* by Donna Lancaster (Penguin Life, 2022)

~ *The Complete Guide to the Menopause: Your Toolkit to Take Control and Achieve Life-long Health* by Dr Annice Mukherjee (Vermilion, 2021)

~ *The Cure for Sleep* by Tanya Shadrick (W&N, 2022)

~ *The Diet Myth: The Real Science Behind What We Eat* by Tim Spector (W&N, 2020)

~ *The Happiness Curve: Why Life Gets Better After 50* by Jonathan Rauch (Thomas Dunne Books, 2018)

~ *The M Word: Everything You Need to Know About the Menopause* by Dr Philippa Kaye (Vie, 2020)

~ *The New Hot: Taking on the Menopause with Attitude and Style* by Meg Mathews (Vermilion, 2020)

~ *The Perimenopause Solution: Take Control of Your Hormones Before They Take Control of You* by Dr Shahzadi Harper and Emma Bardwell (Vermilion, 2021)
~ *Untamed* by Glennon Doyle (The Dial Press, 2020)
~ *Why We Can't Sleep: Women's New Midlife Crisis* by Ada Calhoun (Grove Press UK, 2020) (interviews with midlife women in the US – a Gen-X book)

And should you feel this is your time to give back then you could use your newfound midlife time to volunteer for the crisis text line SHOUT. I trained as a volunteer, and you can do it online from your own home in your own hours with excellent clinical support. SHOUT helps those in a time of extreme crisis via text (mostly under-25s) and relies on an army of midlife women for support. I found it hard, but very rewarding: giveusashout.org/getinvolved/volunteer

Thank-yous

Thank you to . . .

My family for being patient and loving while I wrote this: James, Sky, Grace, Henry and Mabel (and Pixel the Welsh terrier). Sorry I went a little bonkers there for a while, team.

Thank you to our loyal and caring *Postcards from Midlife* podcast listeners and the supportive members of our private Facebook group, many of whom I interviewed for this book. Thank you for sharing your stories anonymously for me.

And thank you to my podcast co-host, Trish, who has supported me through this process of writing a book, which is not easy.

Thank you, Suzanne, whom I have known since the dawn of time as a friend and colleague, who designed the cover with the inspirational illustrator Amrita, a midlife woman with wonderful chutzpah.

To my agent Robert Caskie and my editor Louise Haines and the lovely, vibrant team at 4th Estate.

And thank you to all my friends, new and old: the midlife lifeline.

Endnotes

1   Joanna Whitehead, '10 things we learned from Davina
    McCall: Sex, Myths and the Menopause', *Independent*
    (13 May 2021): https://www.independent.co.uk/life-style/
    health-and-families/davina-mccall-menopause-documentary-
    channel-4-b1846877.html; Maya Oppenheimer, 'Menopausal
    women wrongly prescribed antidepressants which make
    their symptoms worse, warn experts', *Independent*
    (10 October 2019): https://www.independent.co.uk/news/
    health/menopause-antidepressants-symptoms-worse-
    hrt-shortage-a9148951.html
2   Hannah Devlin, 'Dismissal of women's health problems as
    "benign" leading to soaring NHS lists', *Guardian* (2 June 2022):
    https://www.theguardian.com/society/2022/jun/02/dismissal-
    of-womens-health-problems-as-benign-leading-to-soaring-
    nhs-lists
3   Kate Muir, 'Women have struggled to get help with the
    menopause for decades but it's about to change', *Guardian*
    (6 October 2021): https://www.theguardian.com/

commentisfree/2021/oct/06/women-menopause-change-
hormone-replacement-therapy

4   Andrea Petersen, 'Why so many women in middle age are
    on antidepressants', *Wall Street Journal* (2 April 2022):
    https://www.wsj.com/articles/why-so-many-middle-aged-
    women-are-on-antidepressants-11648906393

5   Ibid.

6   J. Kulkarni, 'Perimenopausal depression – an under-
    recognised entity', *Australian Prescriber*, 41 (3 December 2018),
    183–5: https://www.ncbi.nlm.nih.gov/pmc/articles/
    PMC6299176

7   Vaginal atrophy (VA) is a hideous condition caused by a loss
    of oestrogen, the hormone that keeps your vagina soft,
    supple and moist. Losing this hormone means you can
    endure an itchy, dry, painful vagina, and for some women
    this is so severe it means pain just from sitting down. VA
    affects over 80 per cent of perimenopausal women to varying
    degrees and ruins their sex lives, among other things.

8   Amelia Hill, 'Female doctors in menopause retiring early
    due to sexism, says study', *Guardian* (6 August 2020): https://
    www.theguardian.com/society/2020/aug/06/female-doctors-
    in-menopause-retiring-early-due-to-sexism-says-study;
    'Challenging the Culture on Menopause for Working
    Doctors' report, British Medical Association (August 2020):
    https://www.bma.org.uk/media/2913/bma-challenging-the-
    culture-on-menopause-for-working-doctors-report-aug-
    2020.pdf

9   WBUR's *On Point* podcast: https://www.wbur.org/radio/
    programs/onpoint

10 'Landmark study: Menopausal Women Let Down by
    Employers and Healthcare Providers', Fawcett Society
    (2 May 2022): https://www.fawcettsociety.org.uk/news/
    landmark-study-menopausal-women-let-down-by-

employers-and-healthcare-providers; Andrew Bazeley, Catherine Marren and Alex Shepherd, 'Menopause and the Workplace' report, Fawcett Society (April 2022): https://www.fawcettsociety.org.uk/Handlers/Download.ashx?IDMF=9672cf45-5f13-4b69-8882-1e5e643ac8a6

11 Stephanie Lane, 'The scary facts behind the gender pension gap', World Economic Forum (7 May 2018): https://www.weforum.org/agenda/2018/03/retired-women-less-money-pensions-than-men